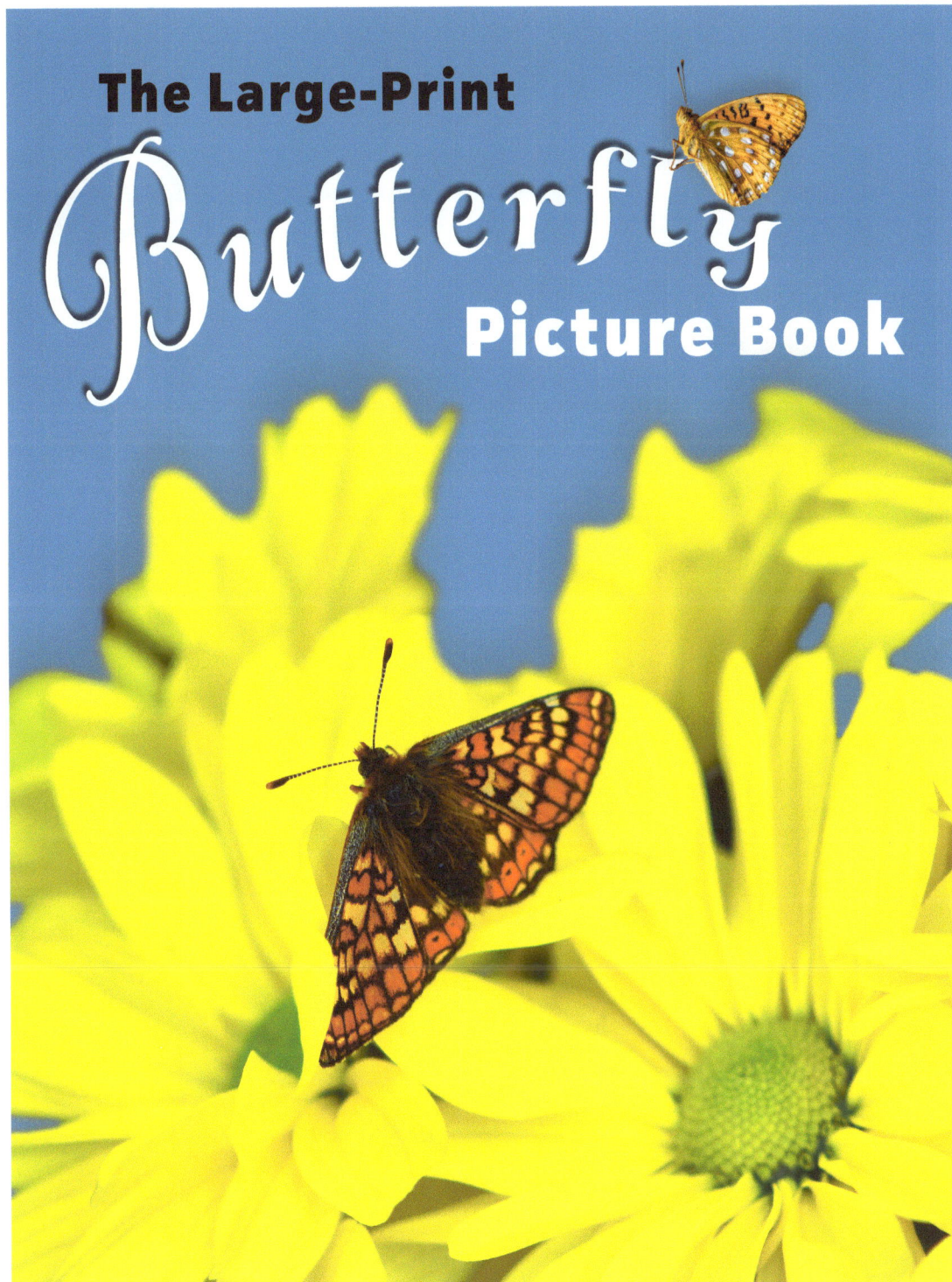

The Large-Print

Butterfly

Picture Book

Copyright © 2020 by Lasting Happiness
ISBN: 978-1-9995487-7-3

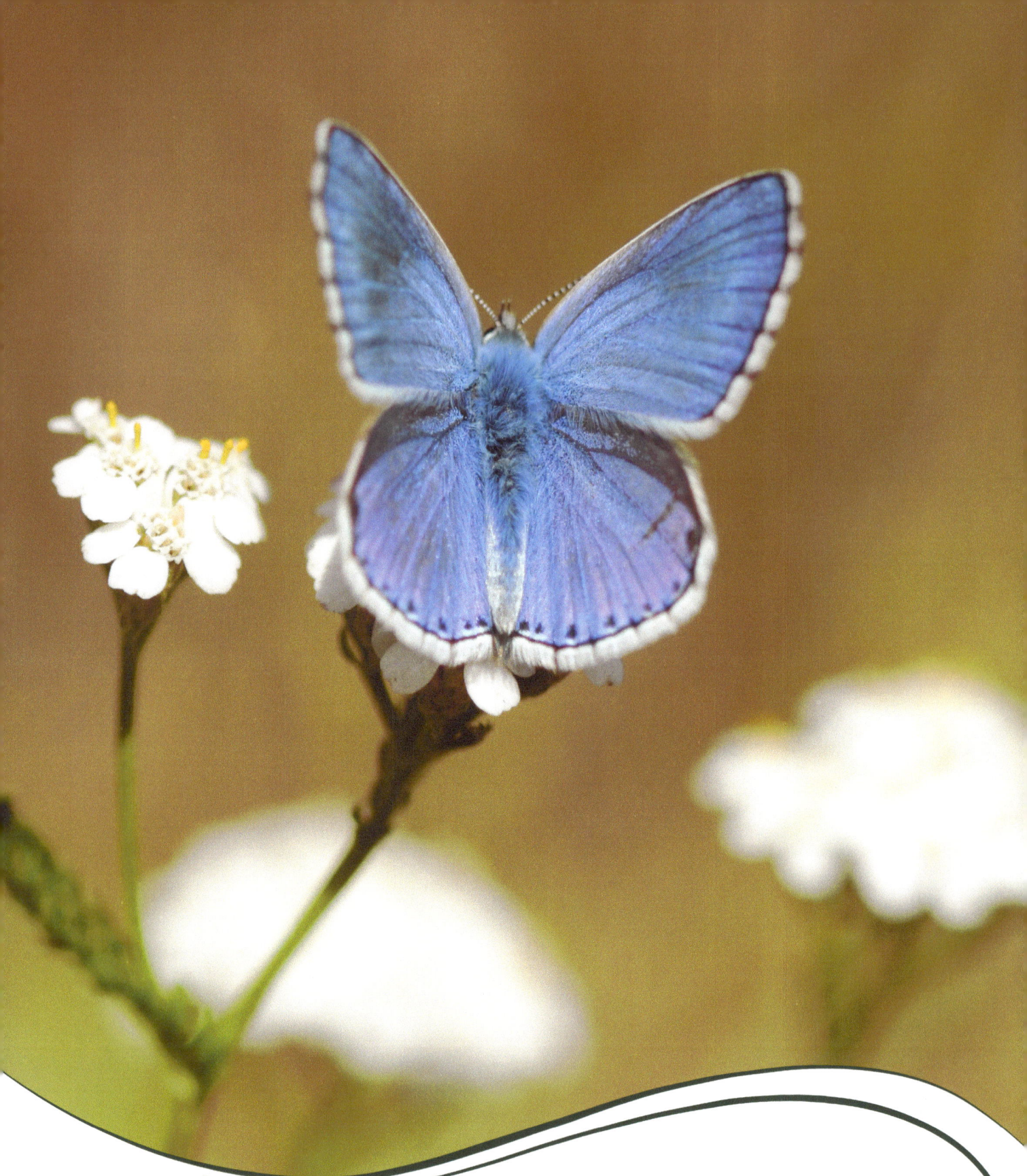

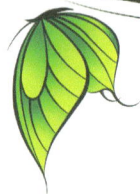

Adonis Blue Butterfly

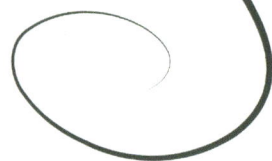

Black Hairstreak Butterfly

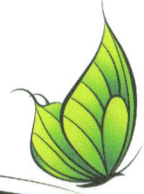

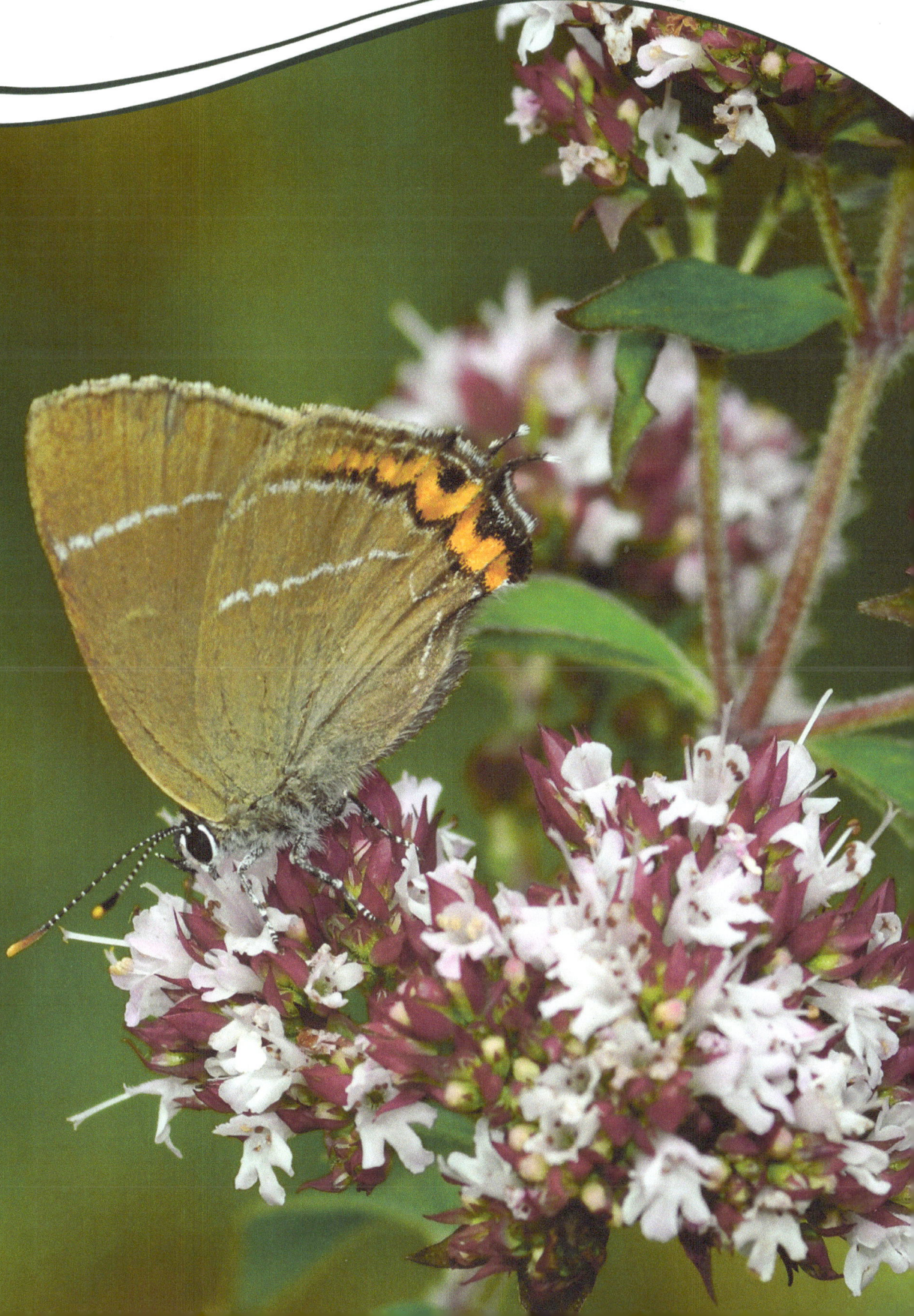

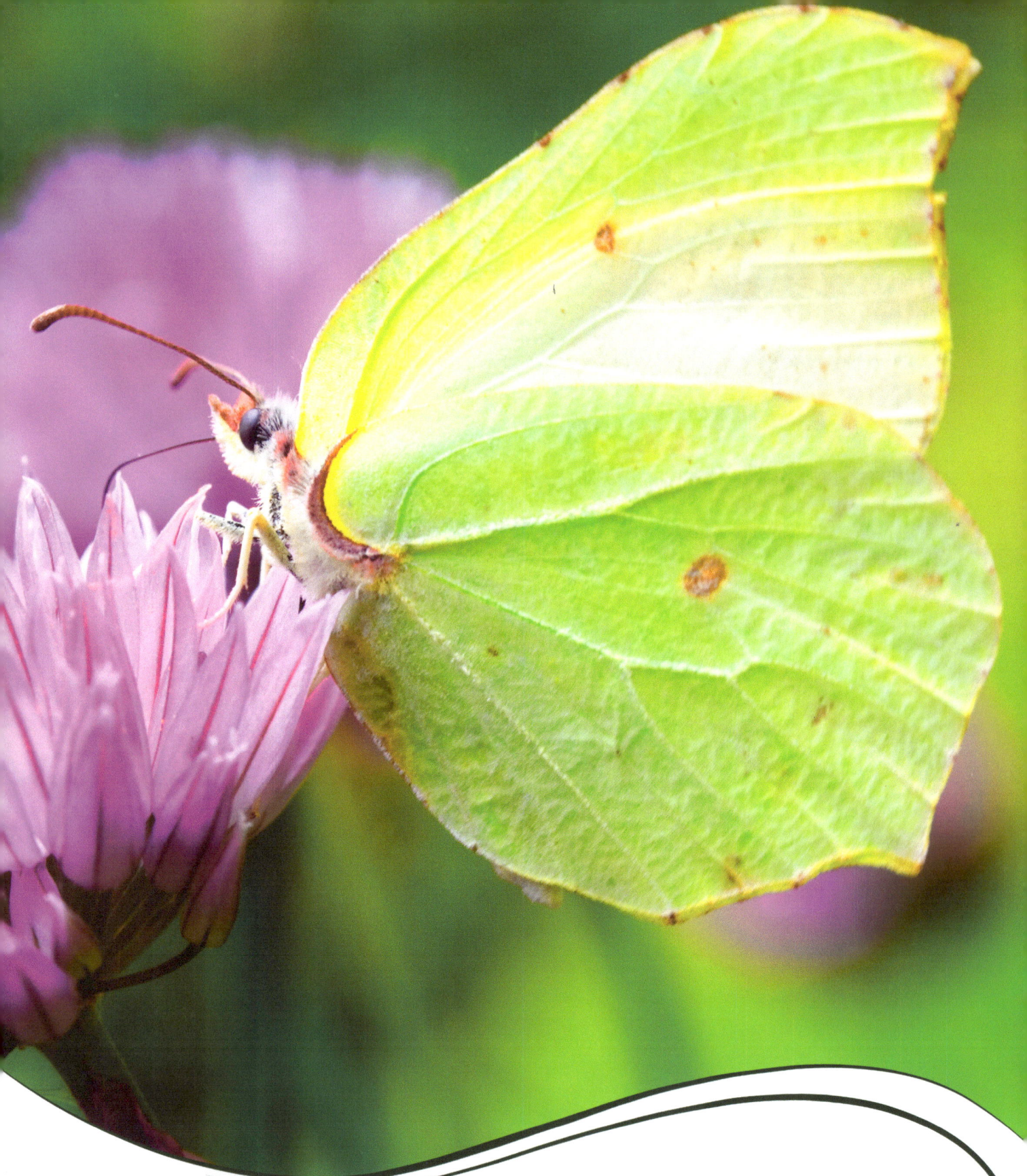

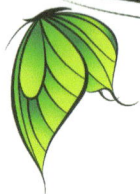

Brimstone Butterfly

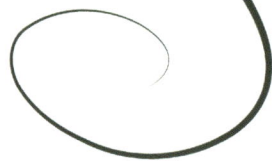

Brown Argus Butterfly

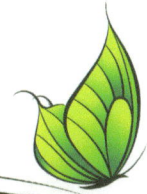

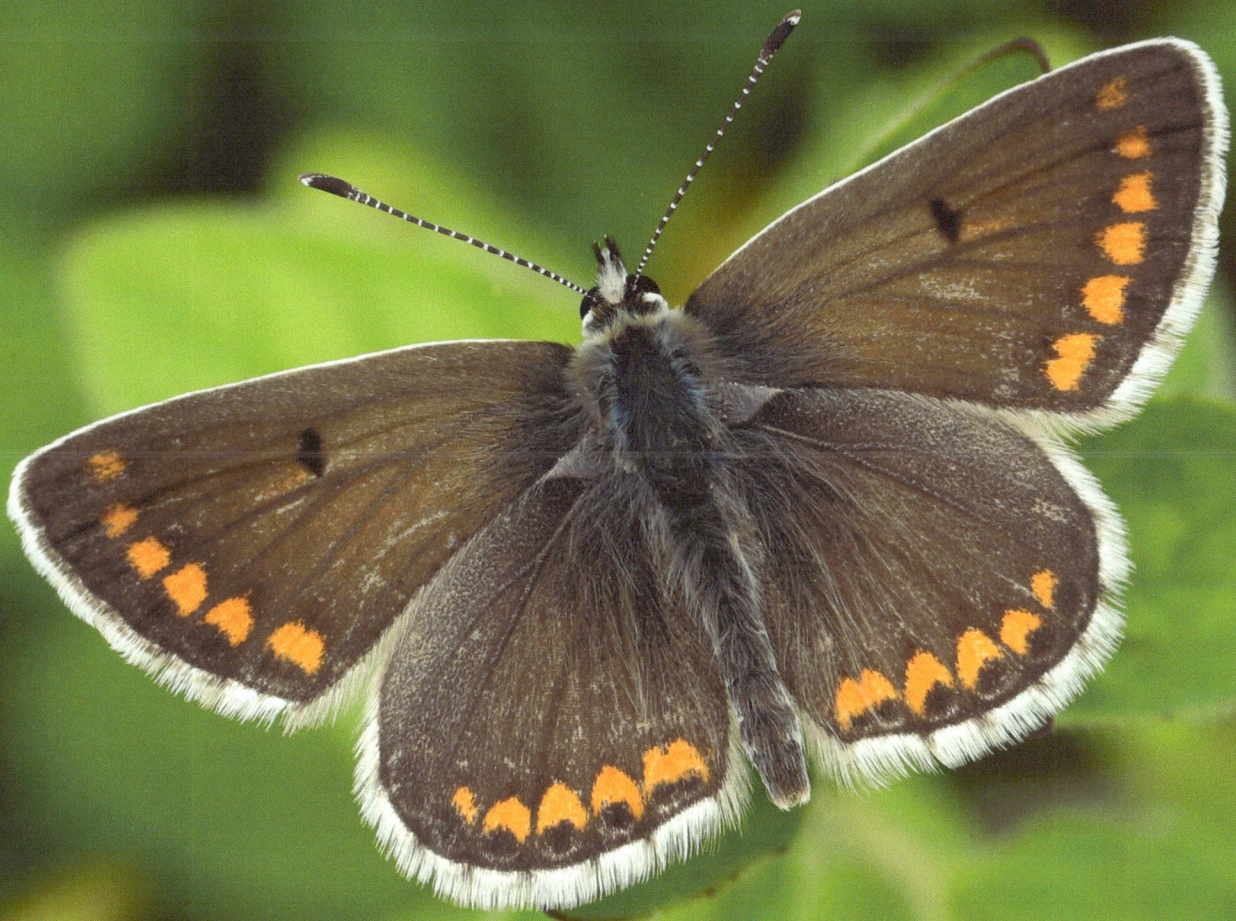

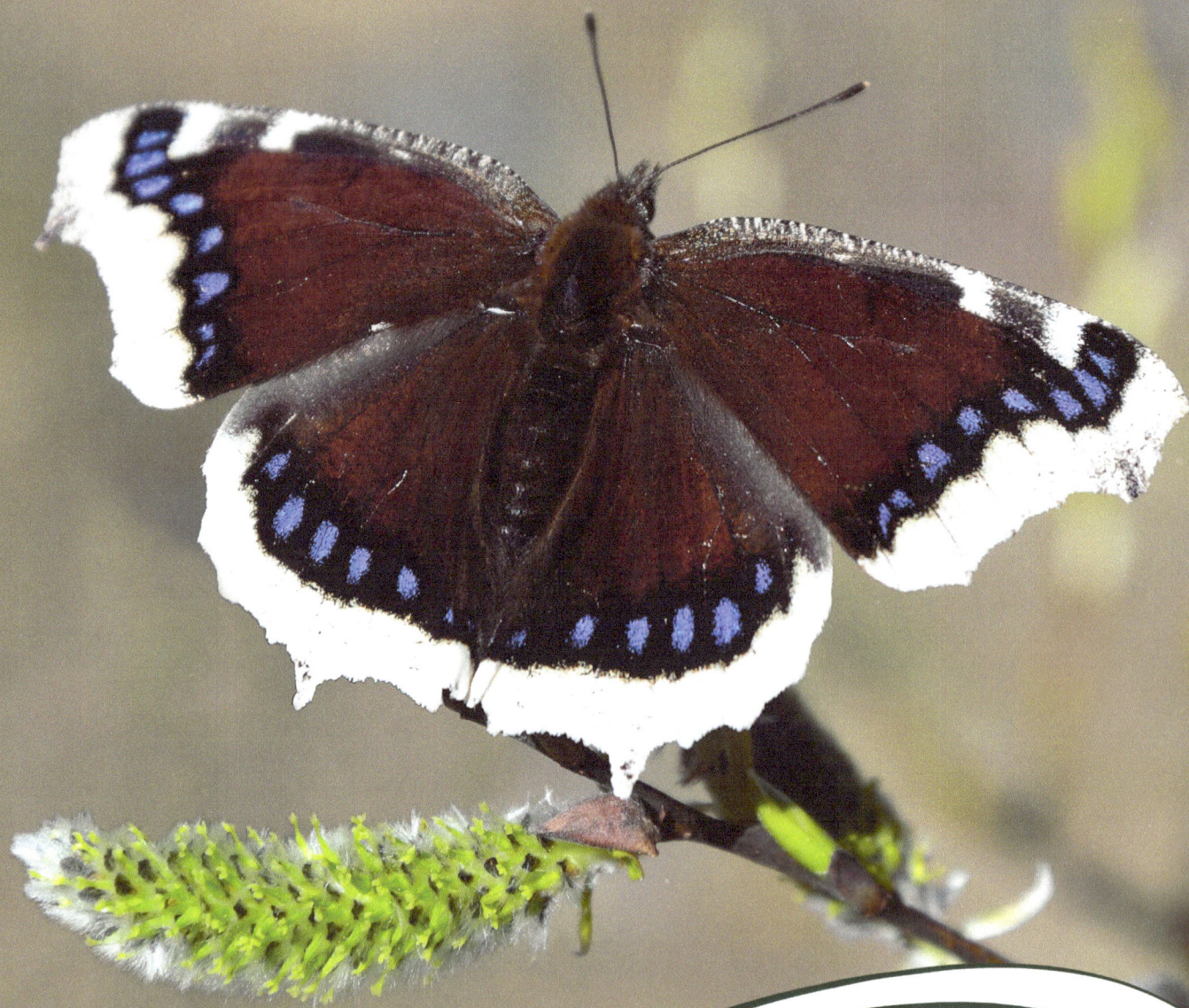

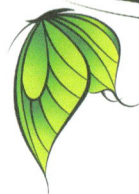

Camberwell Beauty Butterfly

Chalk Hill Blue Butterfly

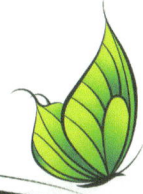

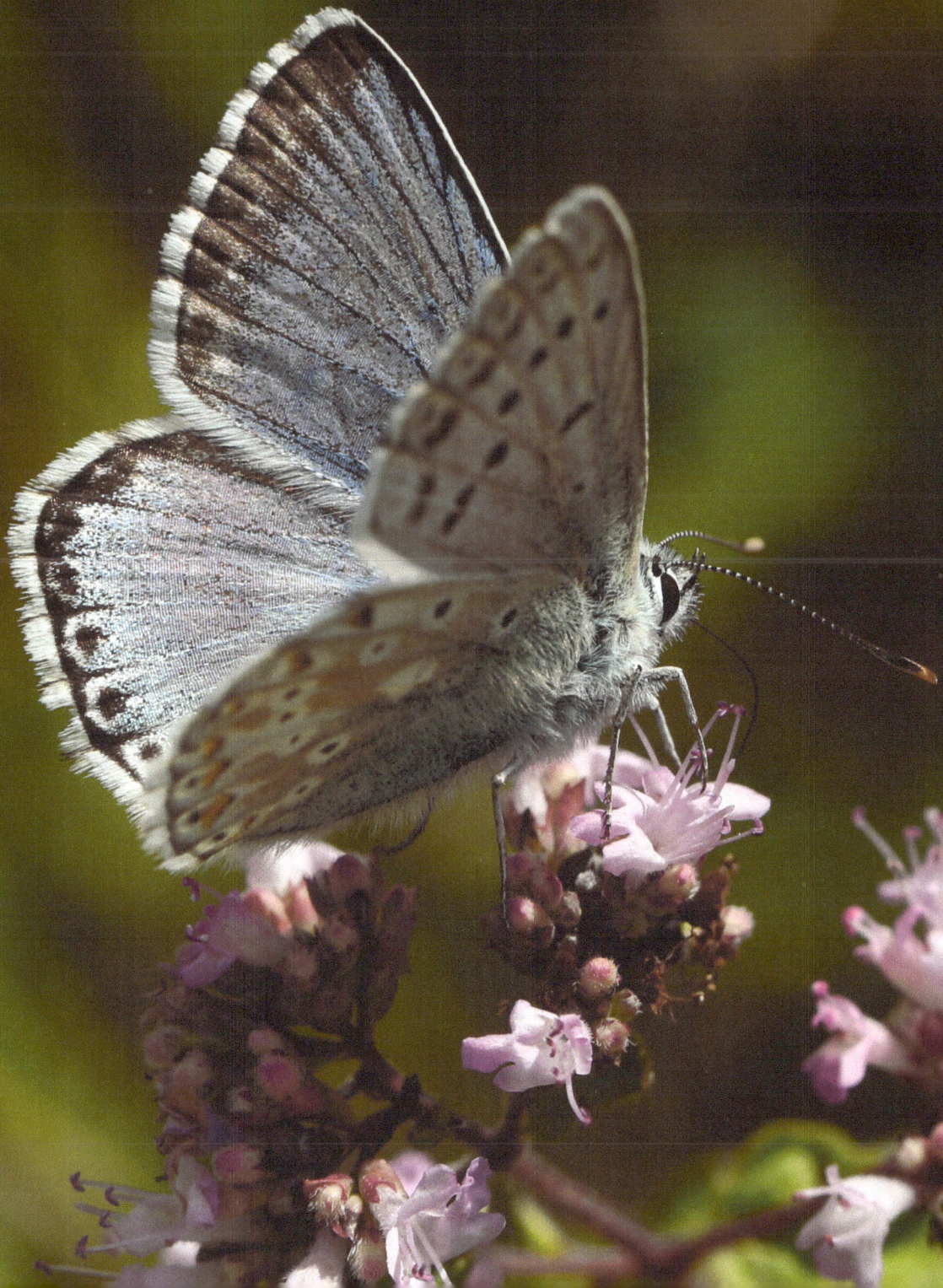

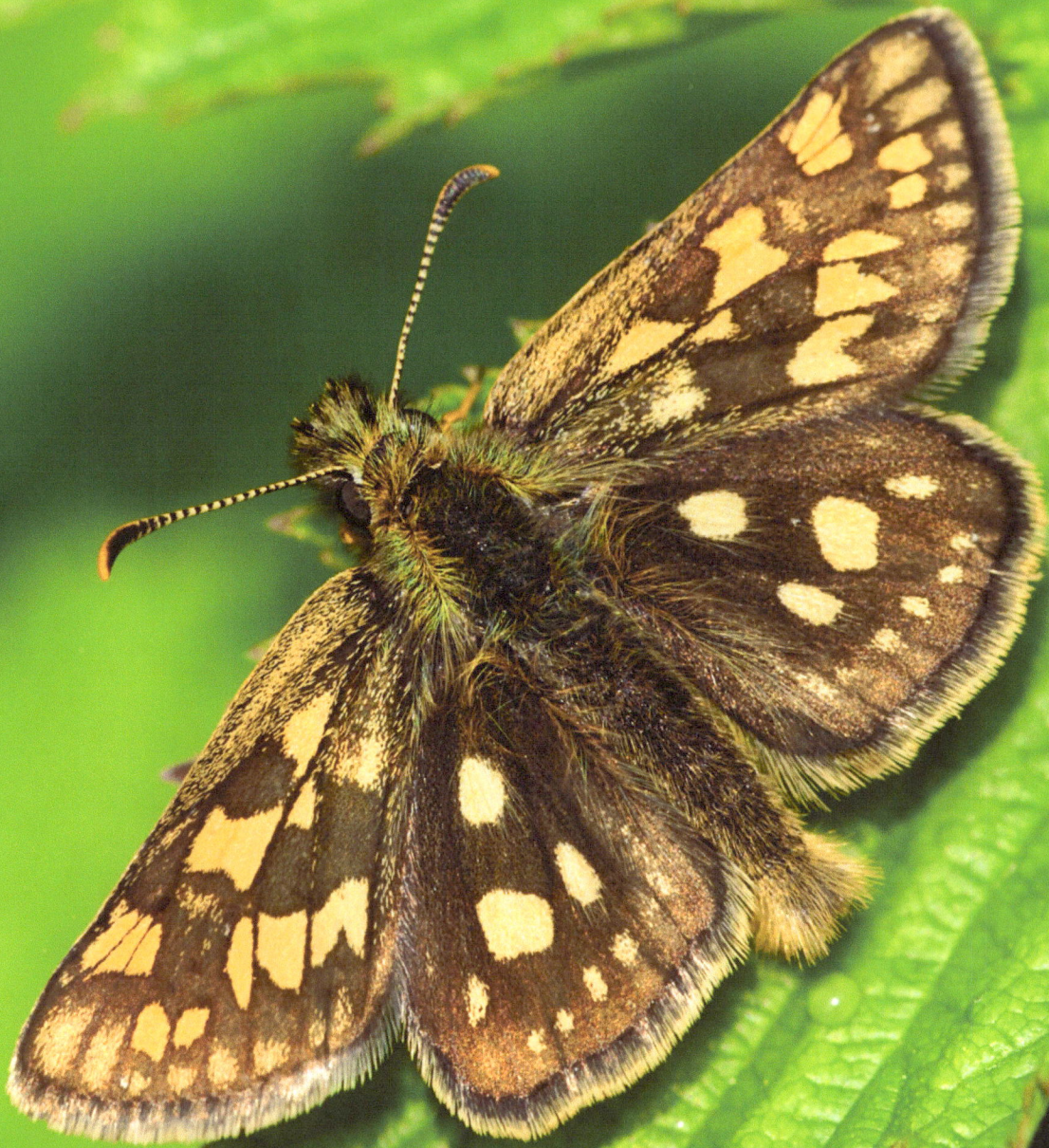

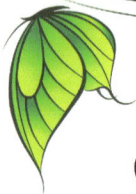

Chequered Skipper Butterfly

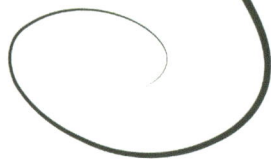

Clouded Yellow Butterfly

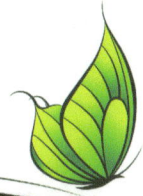

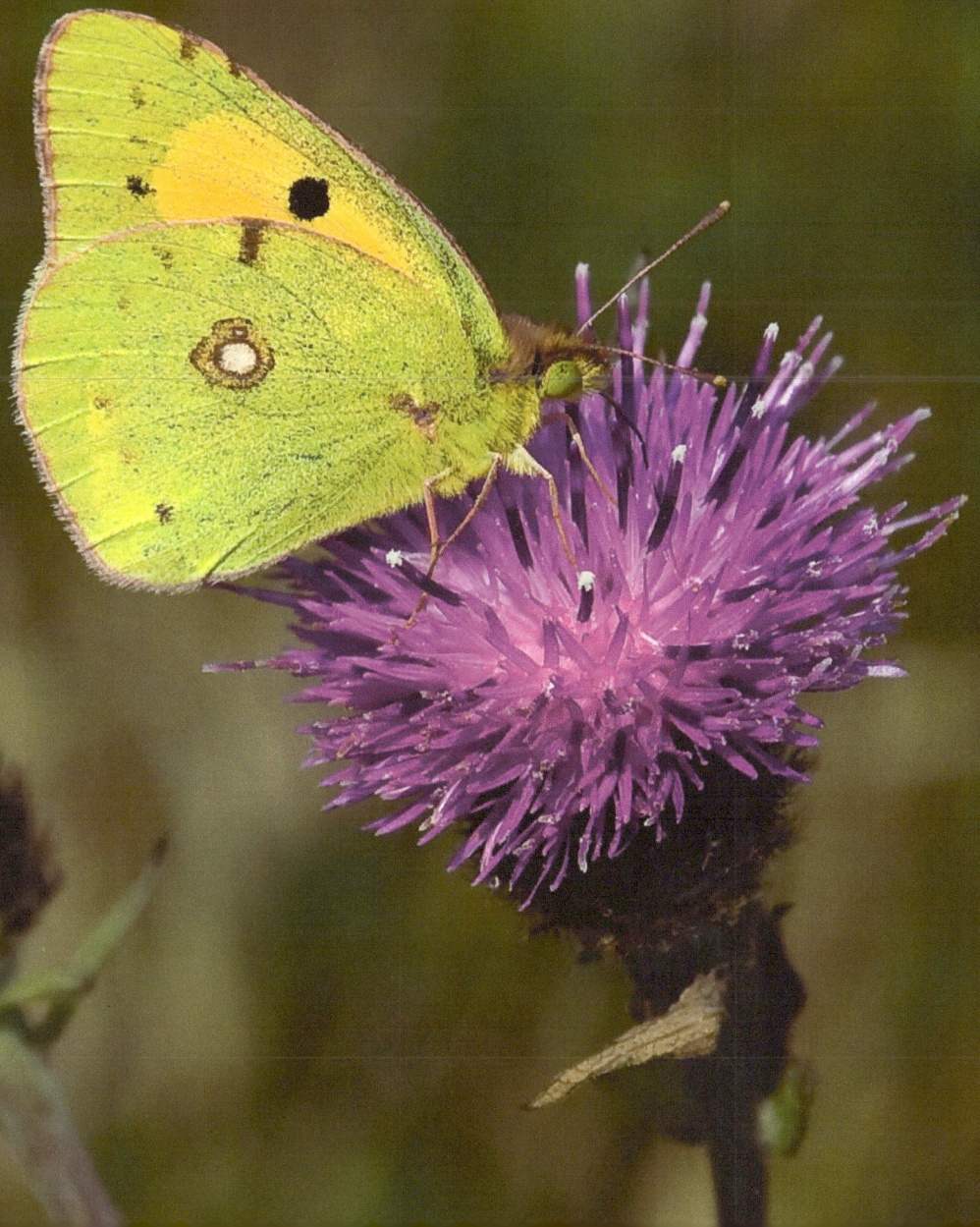

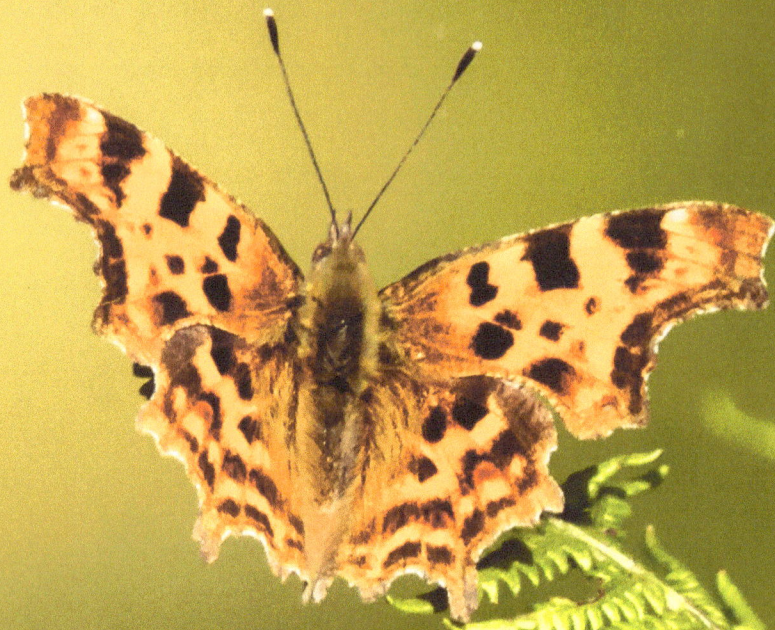

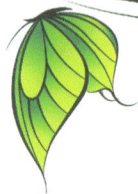

Comma
Butterfly

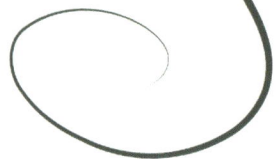

Common Blue Butterfly

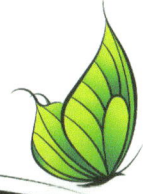

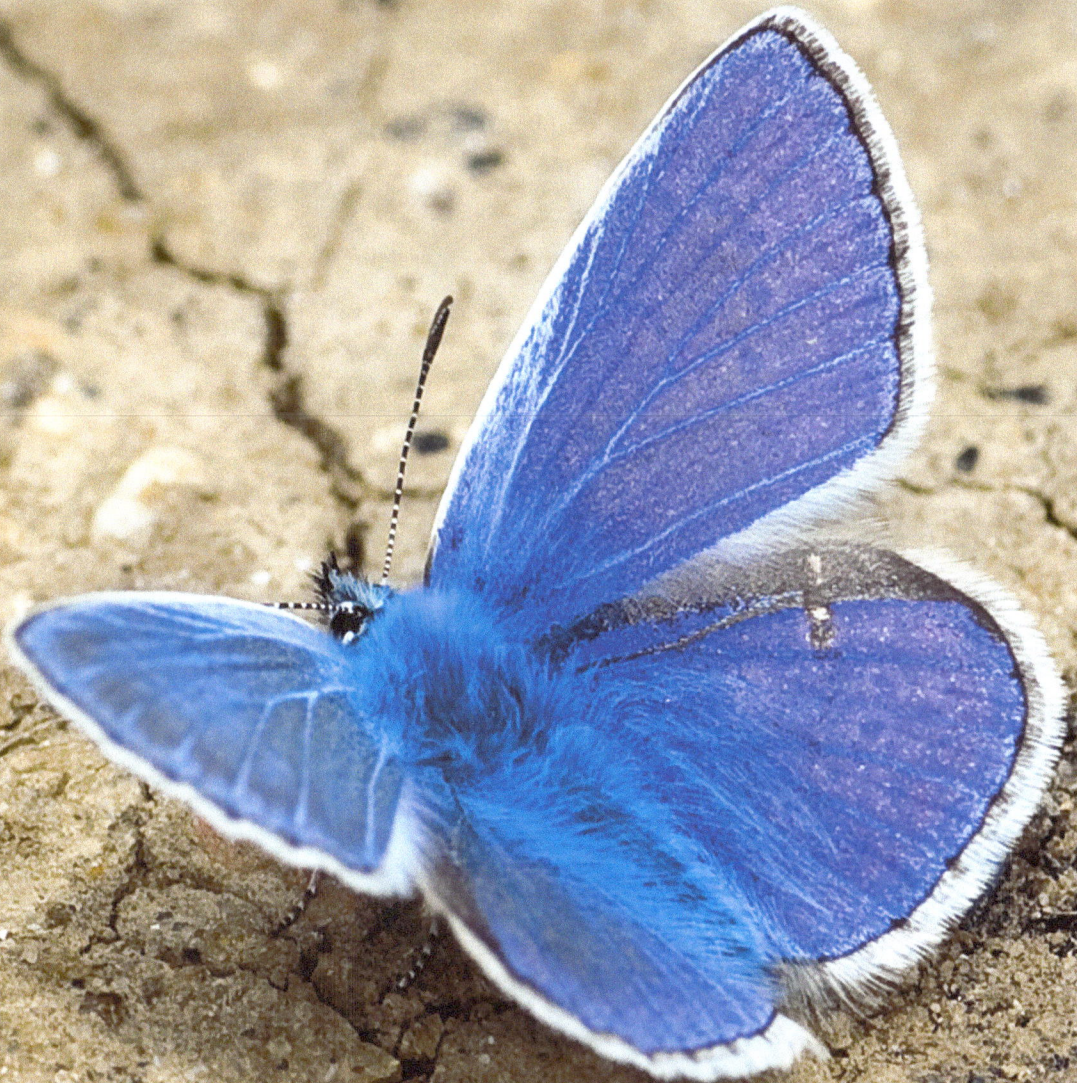

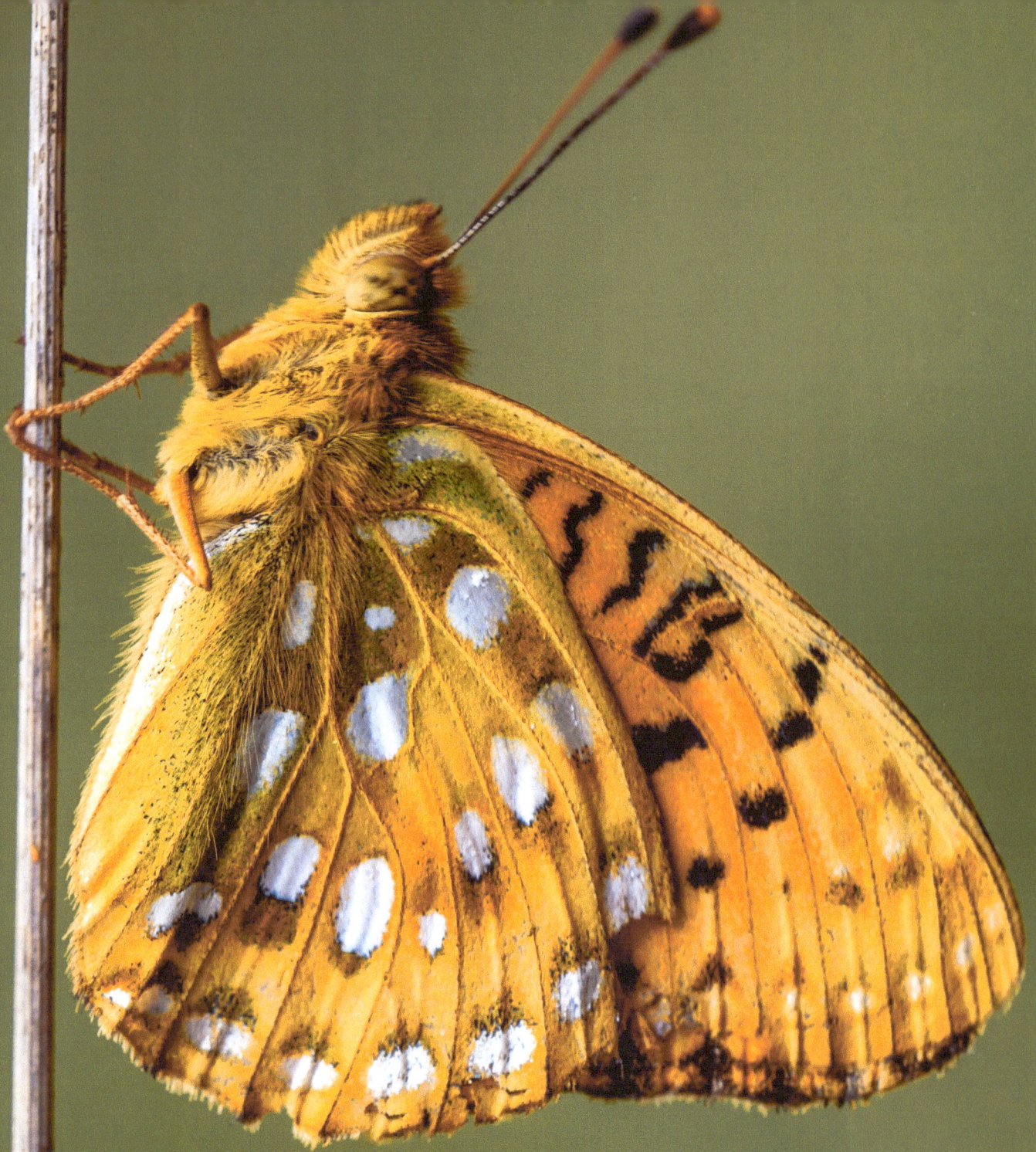

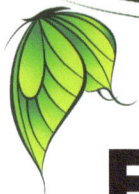

Dark Green
Fritillary Butterfly

Dingy Skipper Butterfly

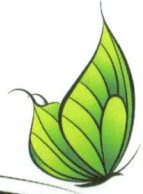

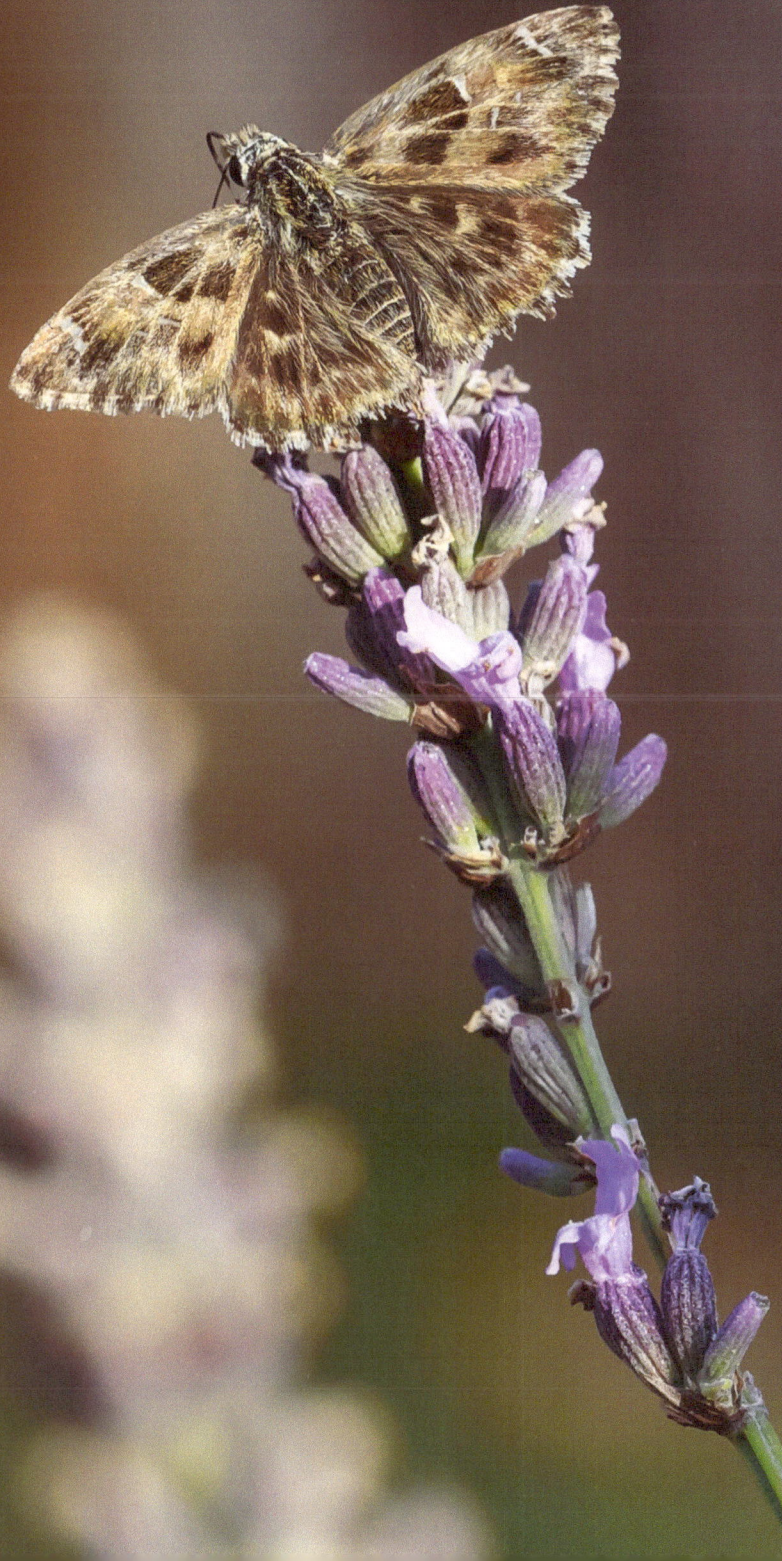

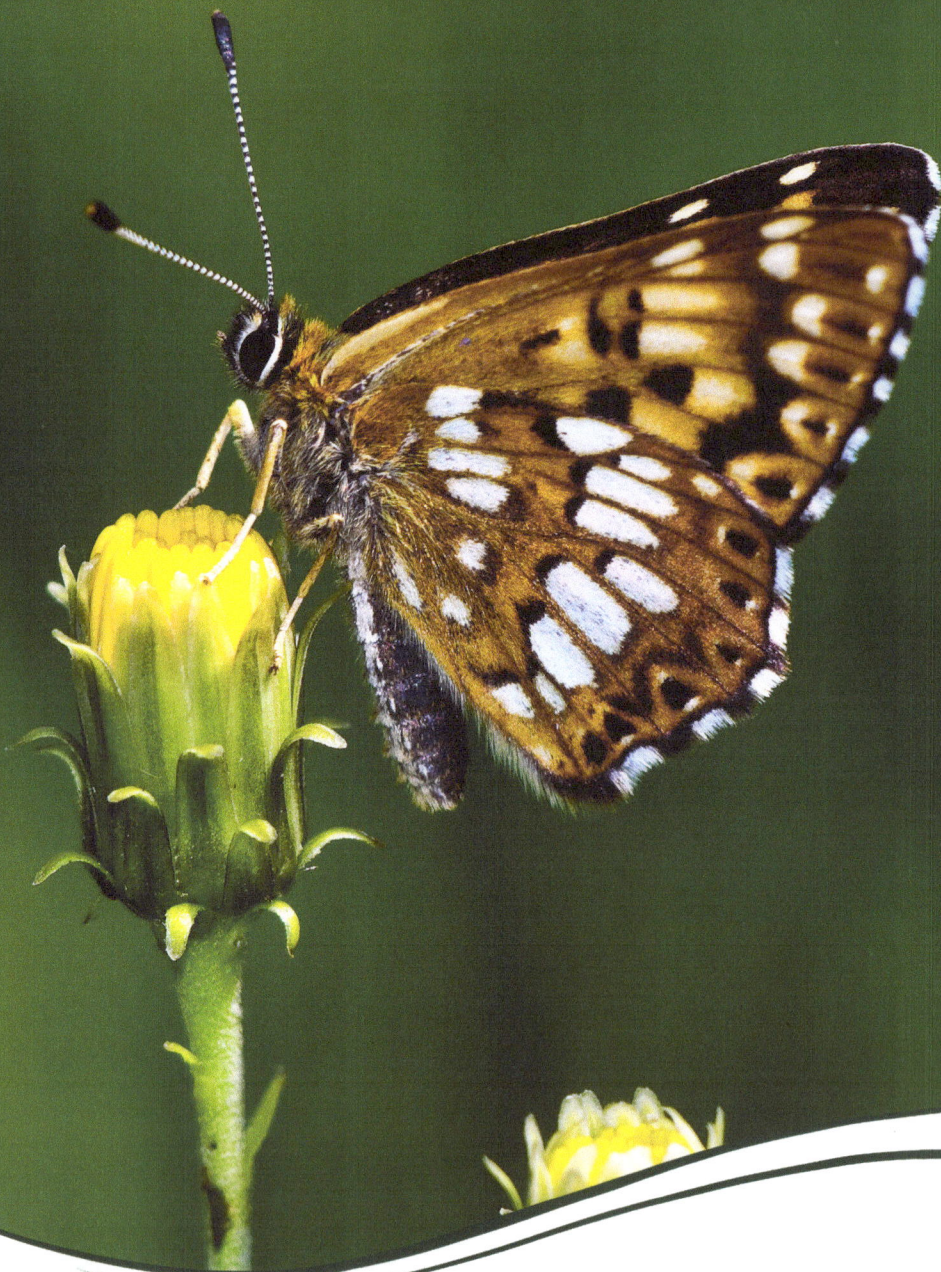

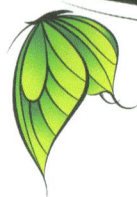

Duke of Burgundy Butterfly

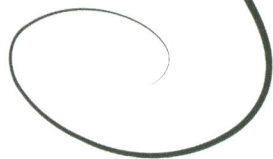

Essex Skipper Butterfly

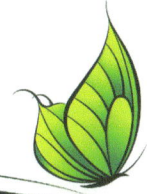

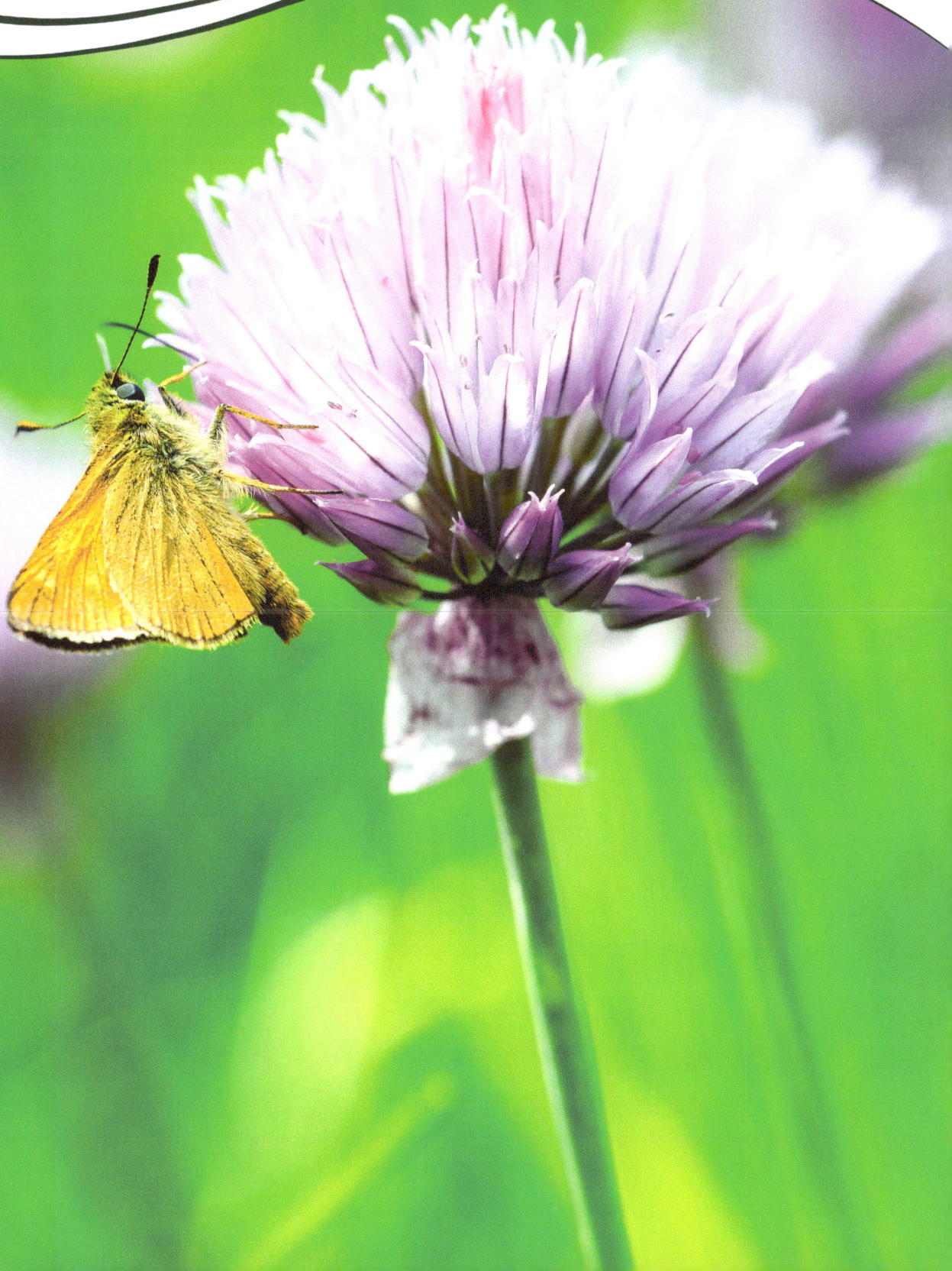

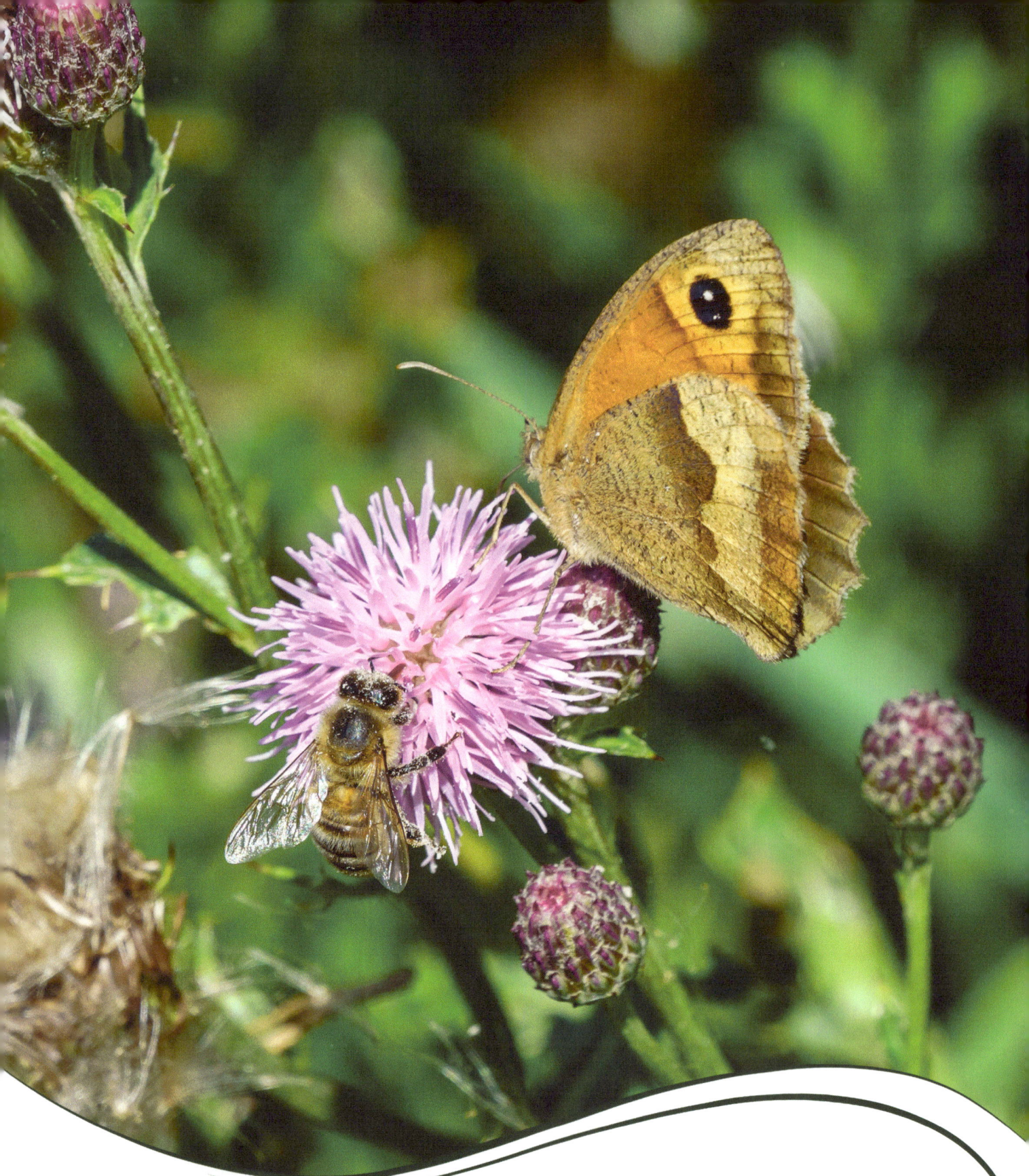

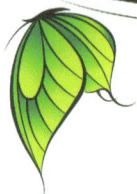

Gatekeeper
Butterfly

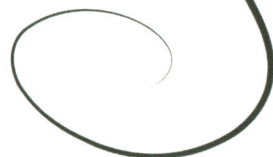

Glanville Fritillary Butterfly

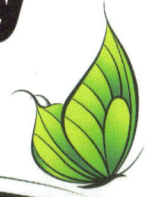

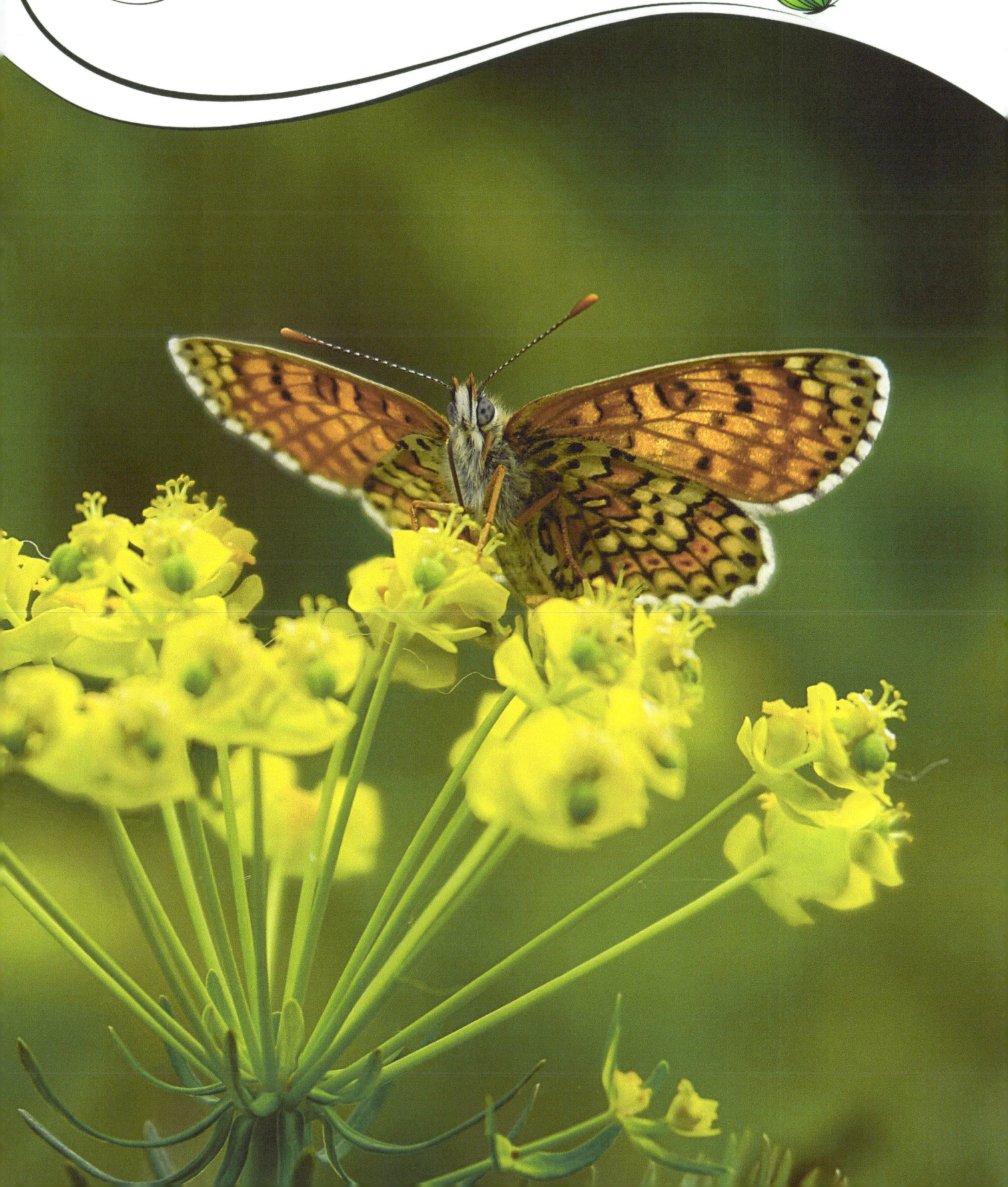

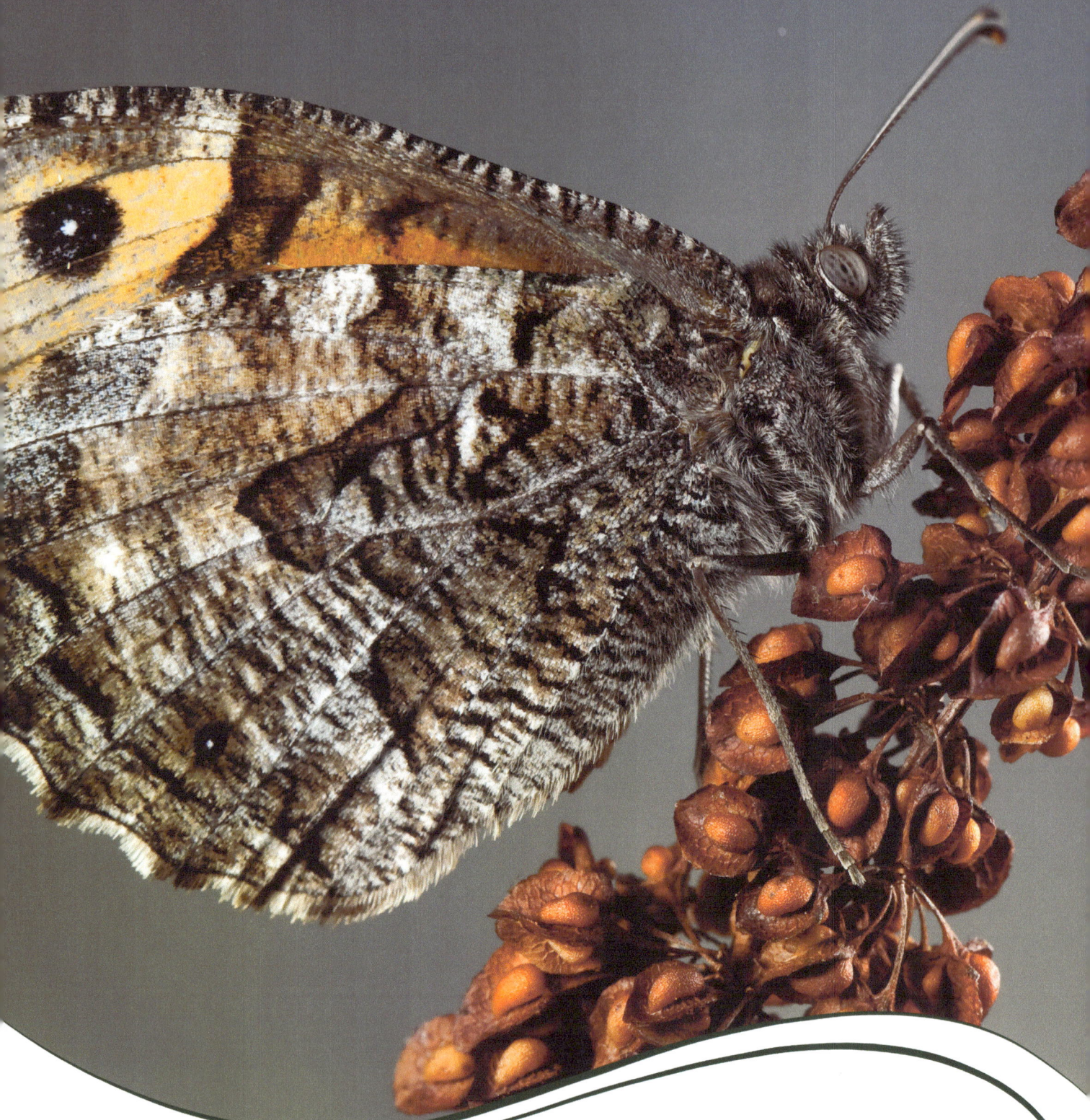

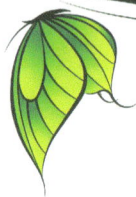

Grayling
Butterfly

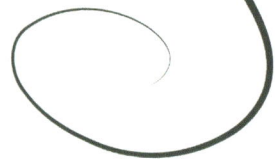

Green Hairstreak Butterfly

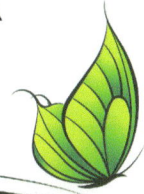

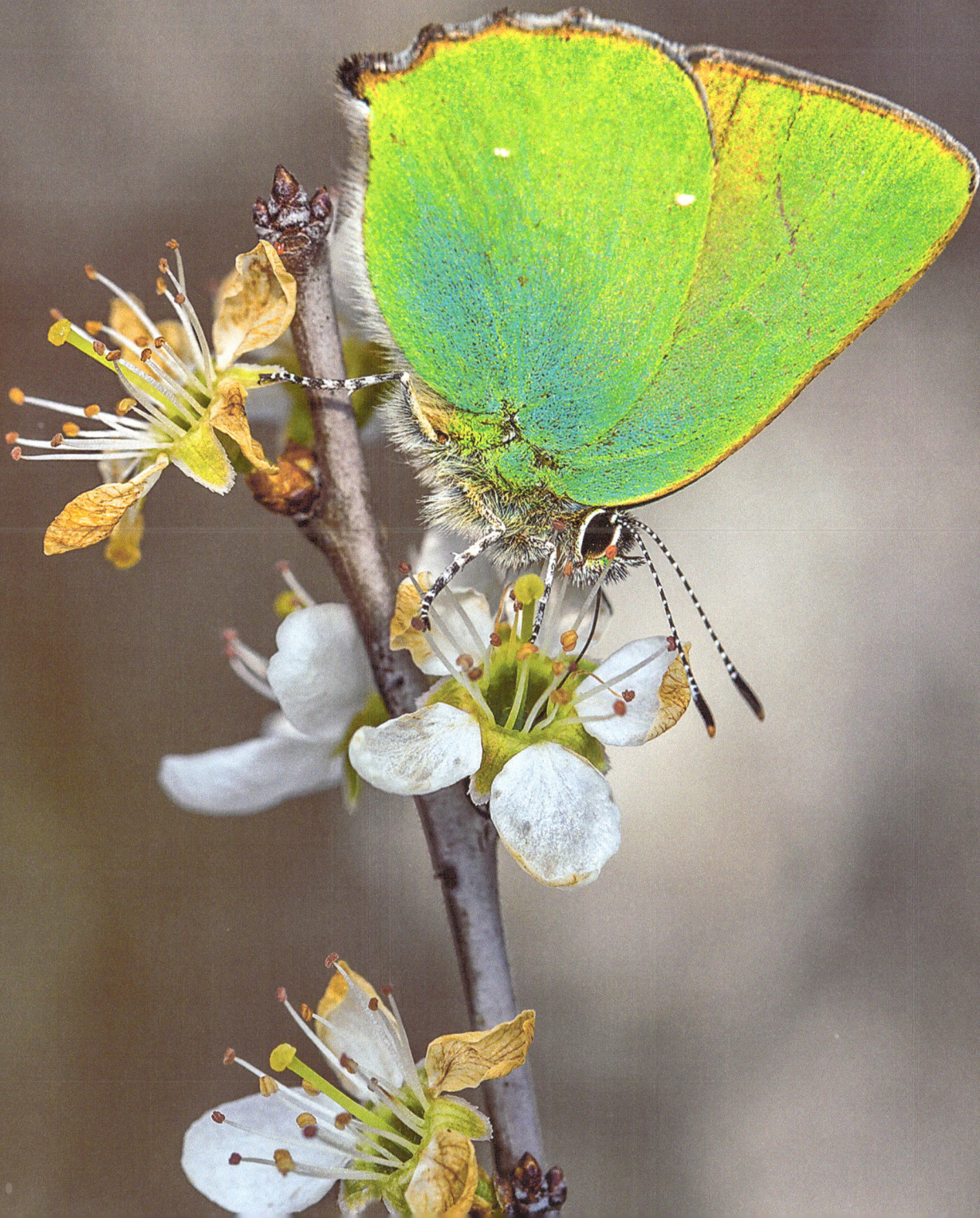

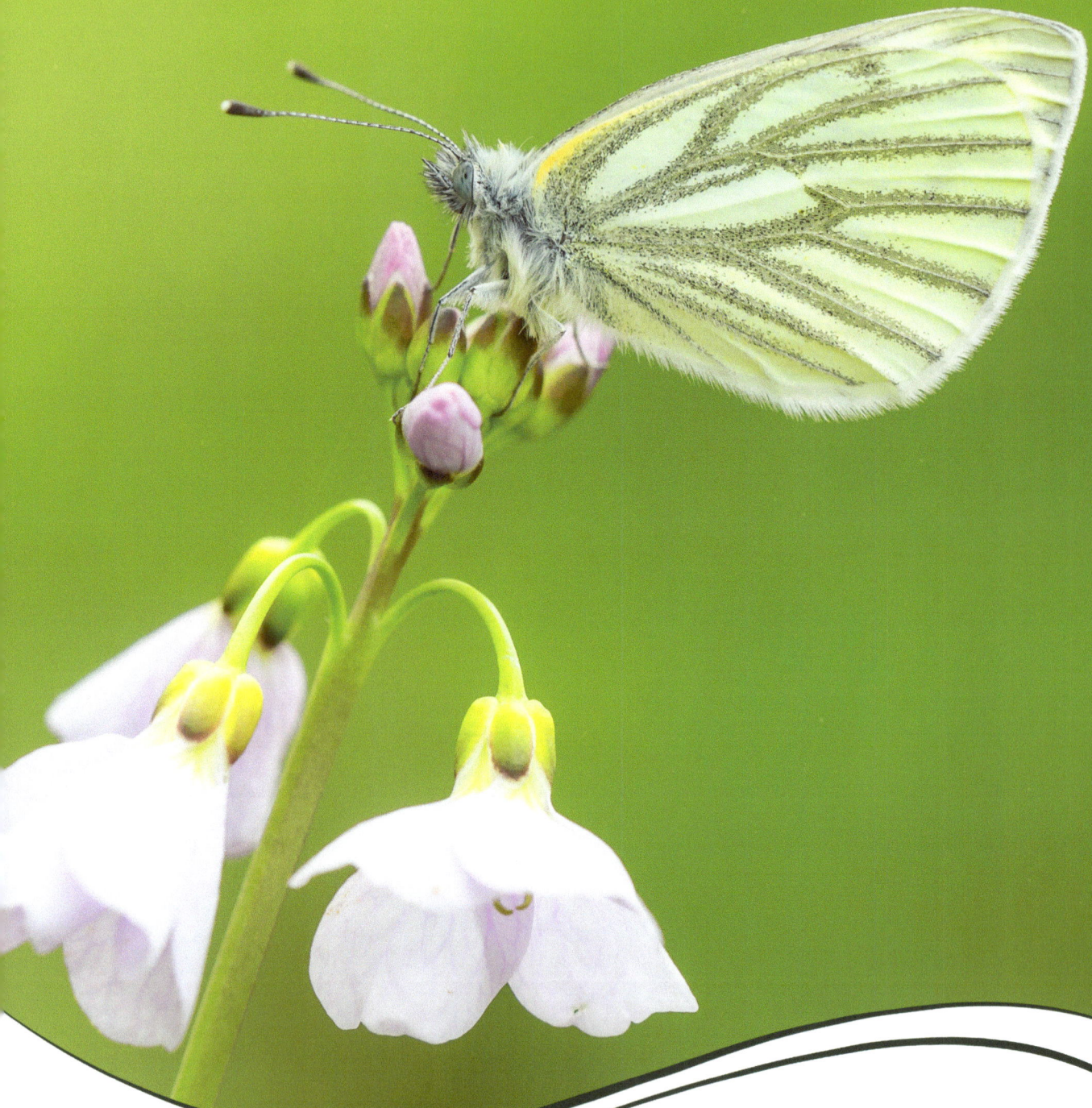

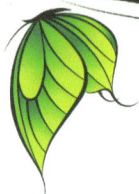

Green-veined White Butterfly

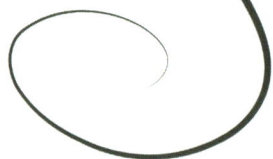

Grizzled Skipper Butterfly

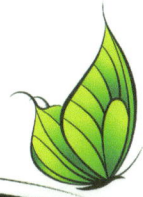

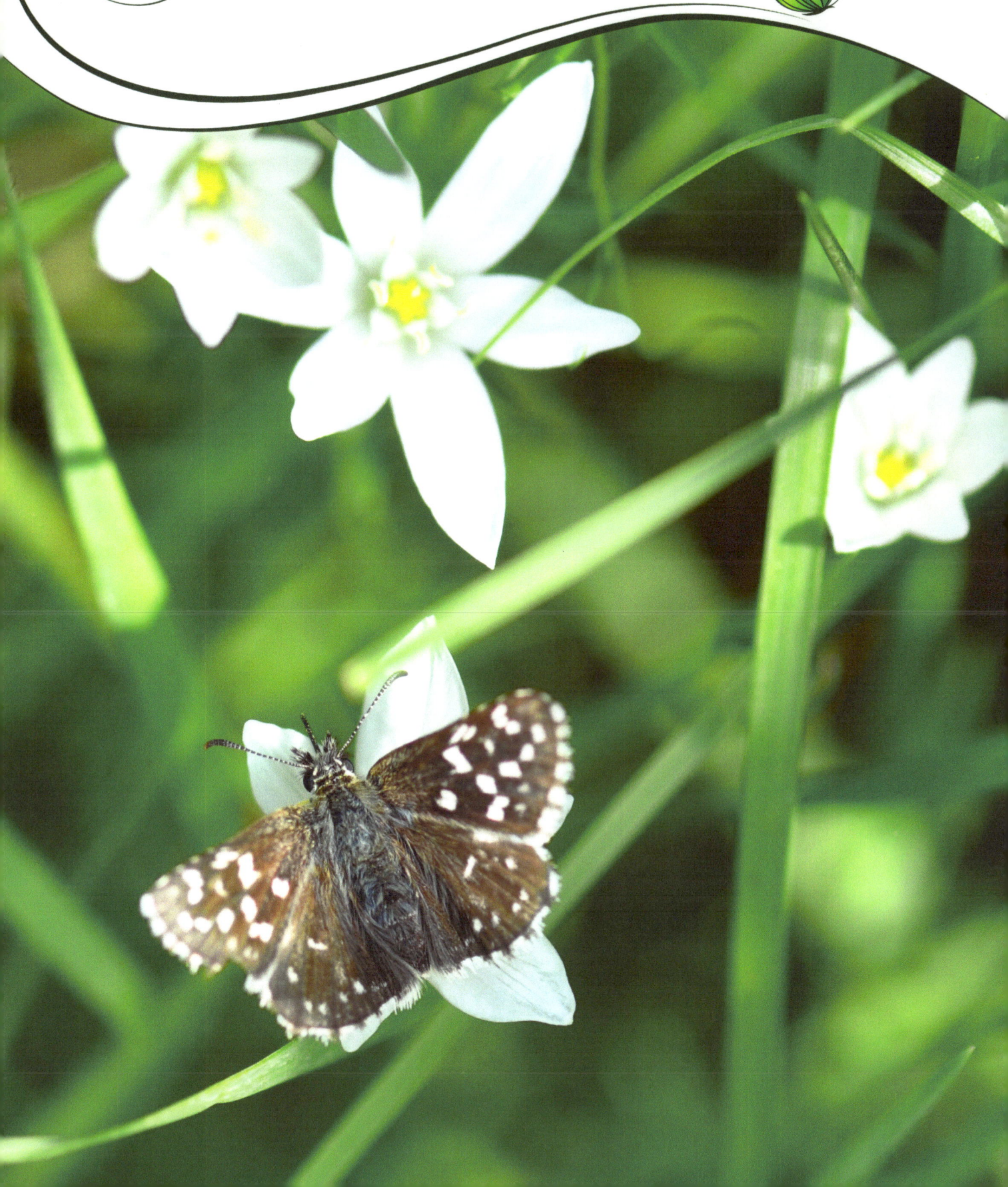

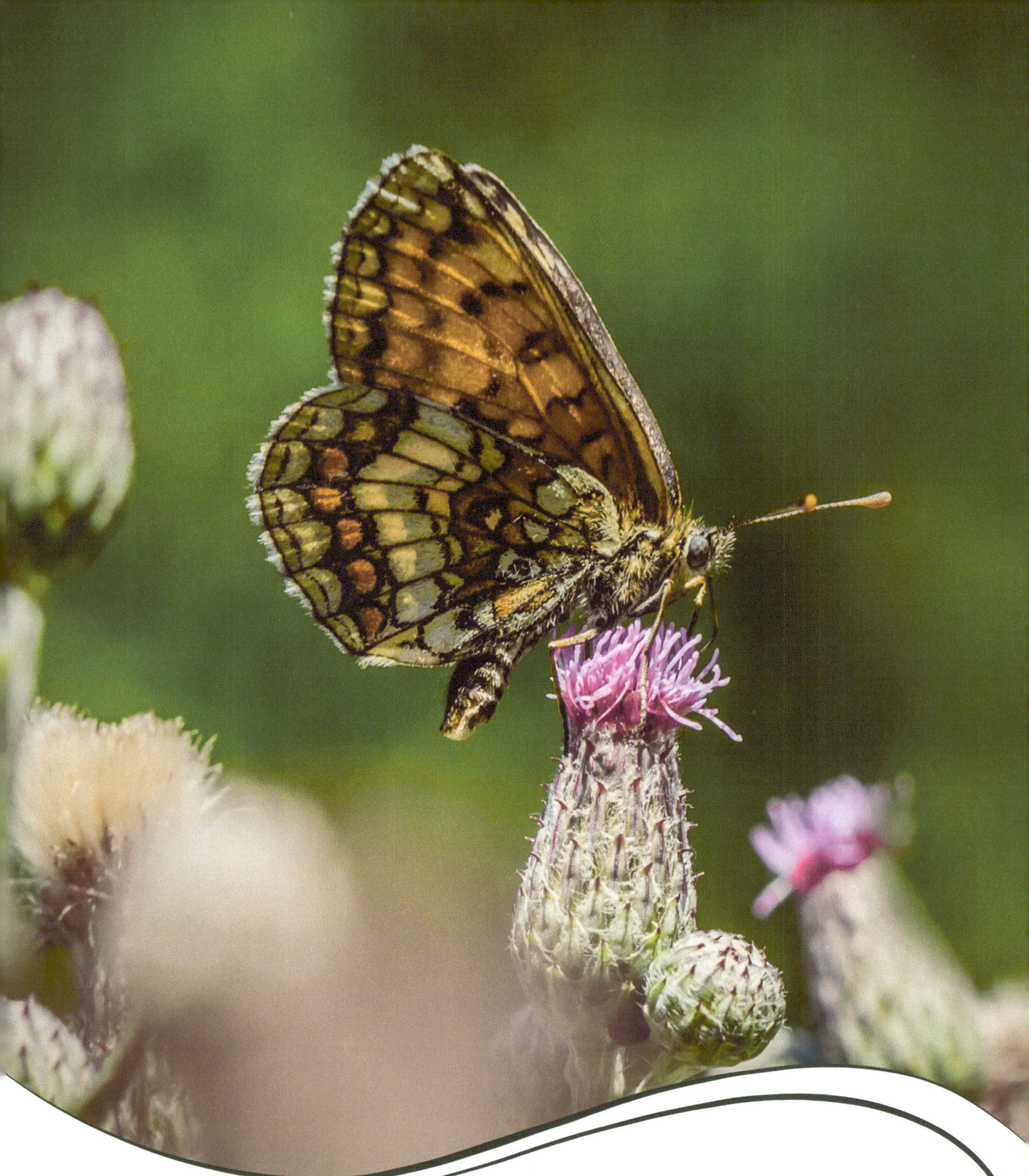

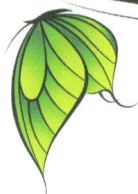

Heath Fritillary
Butterfly

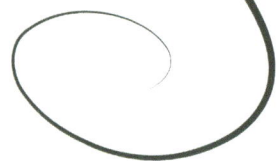

High Brown Fritillary Butterfly

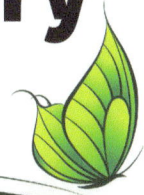

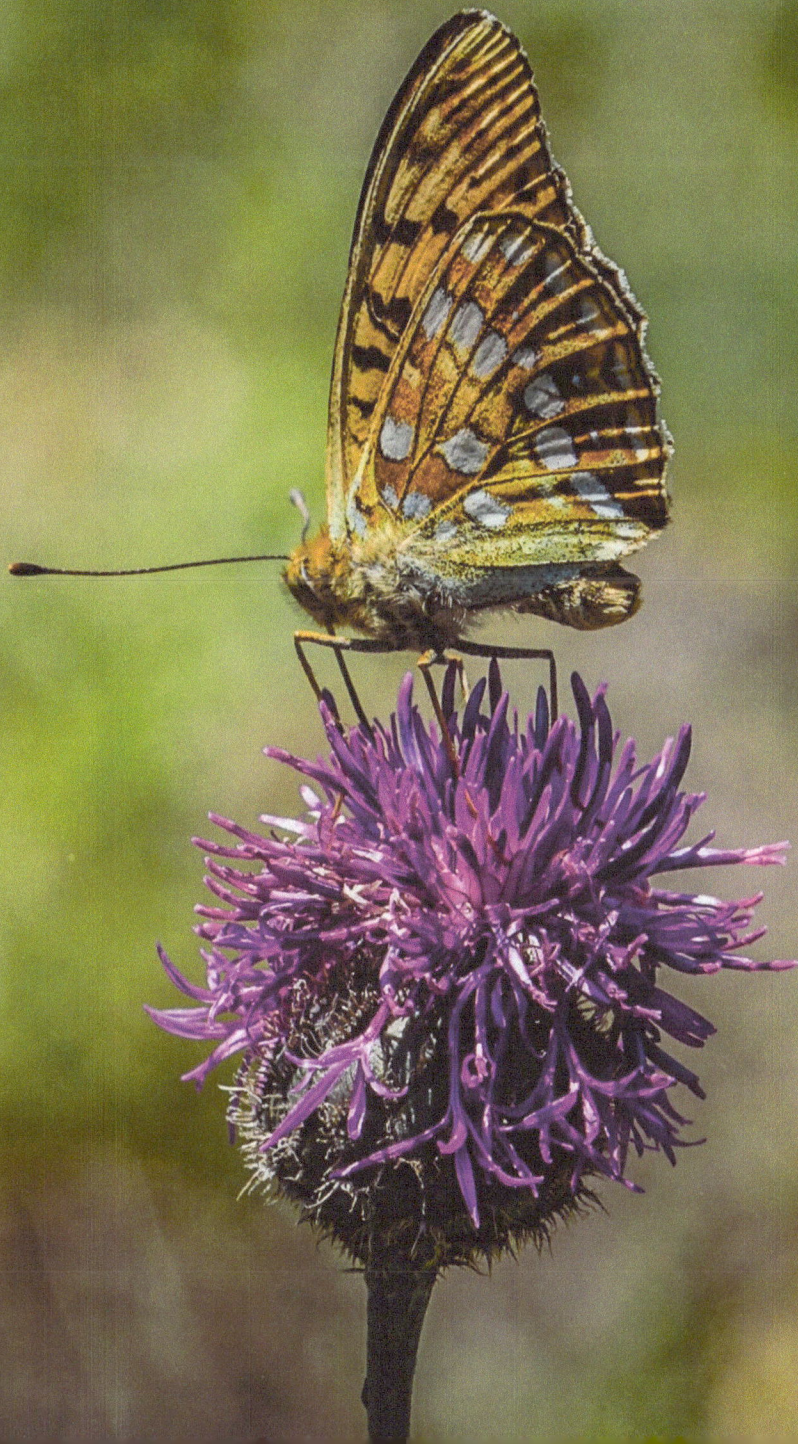

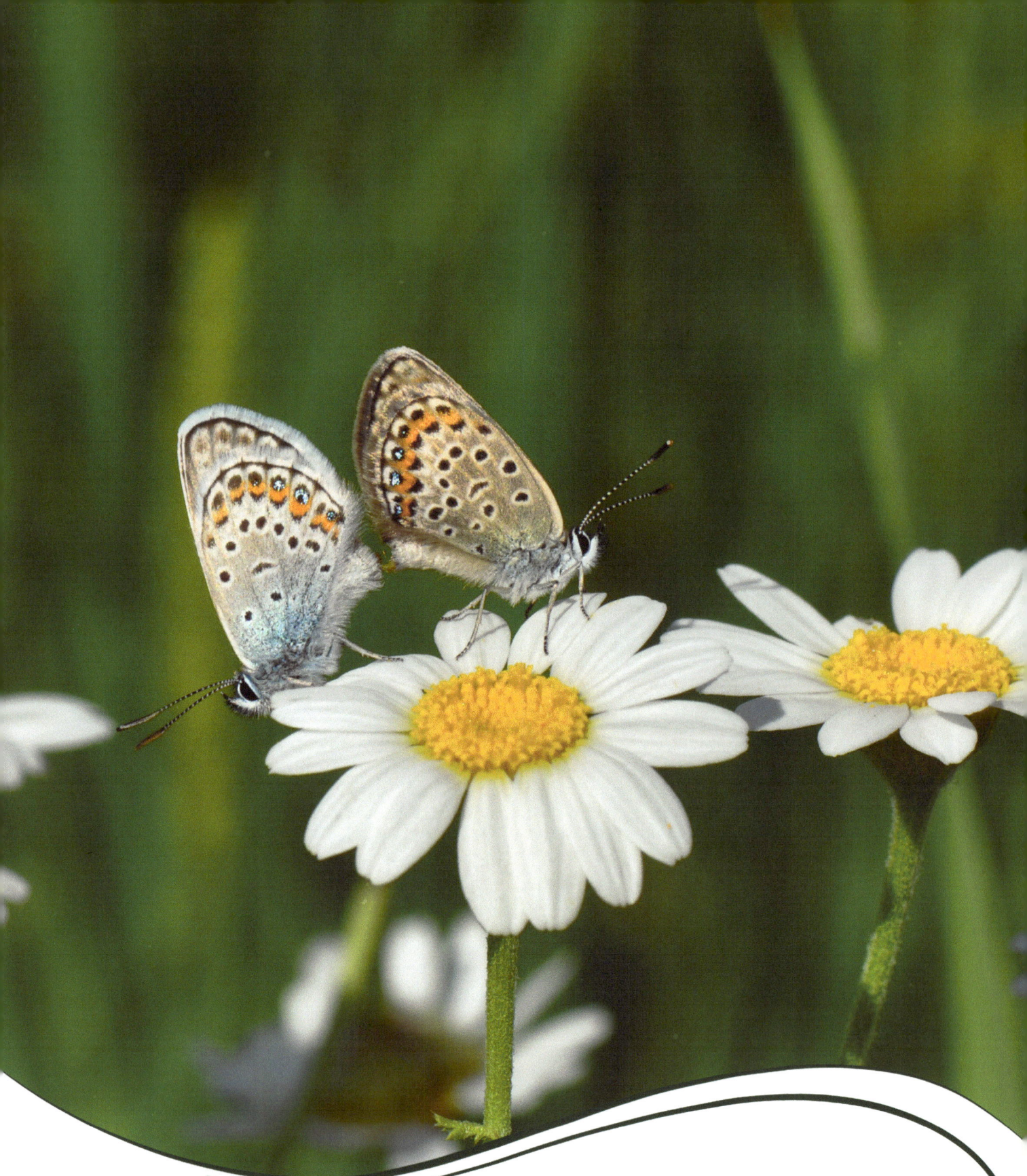

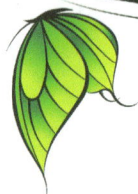

Large Blue Butterfly

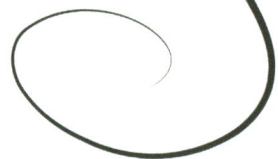

Large Copper Butterfly

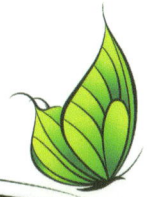

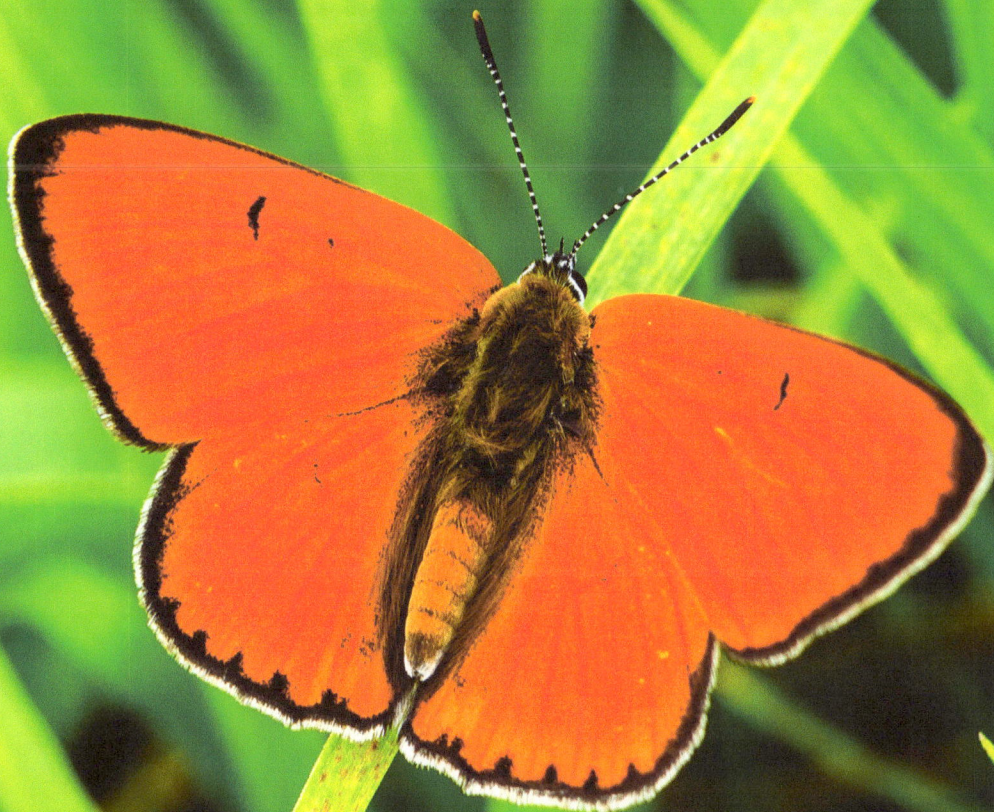

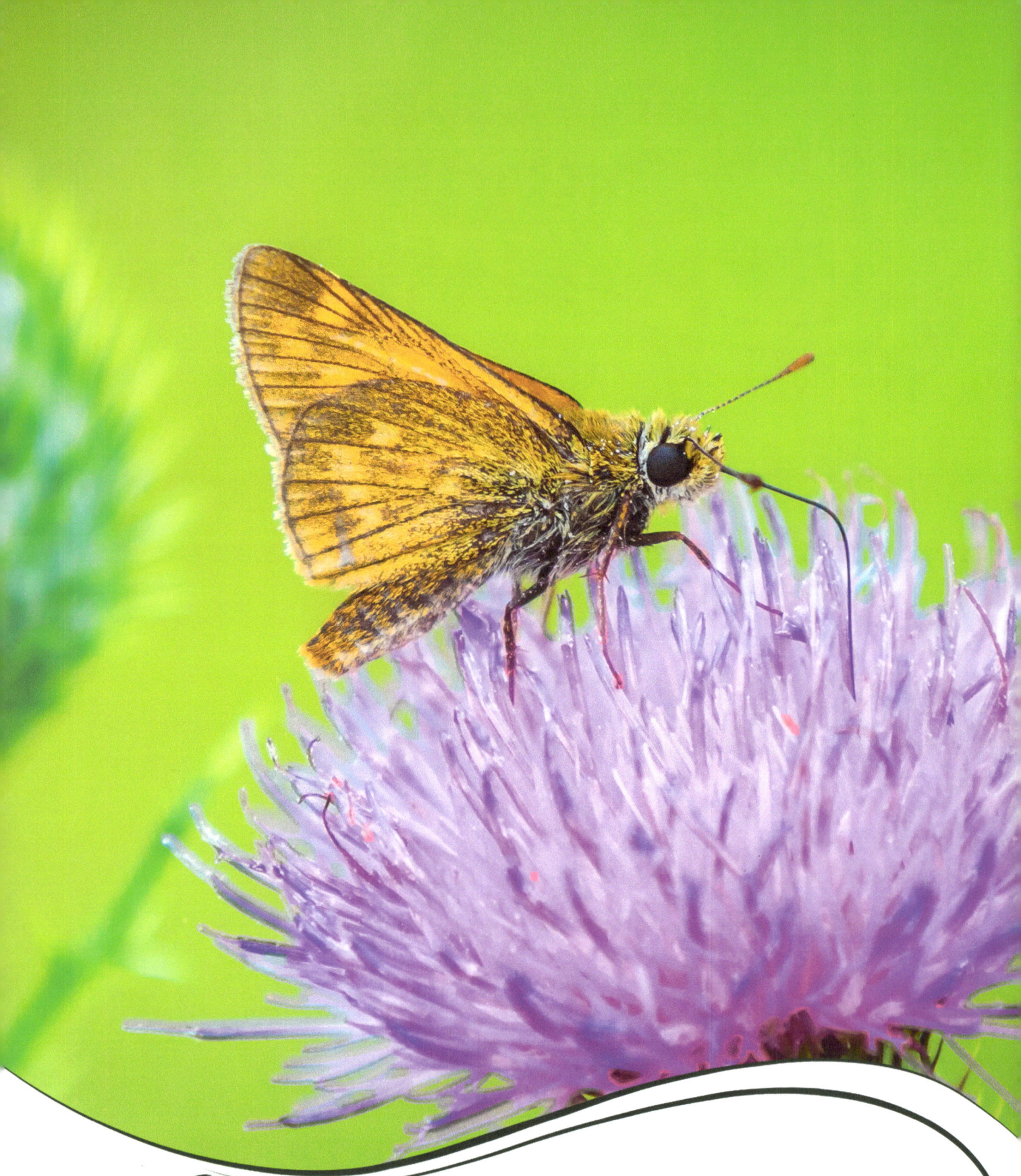

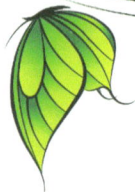

Large Skipper Butterfly

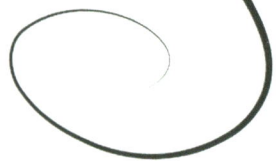

Large Tortoiseshell Butterfly

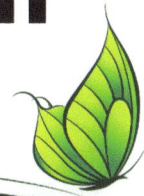

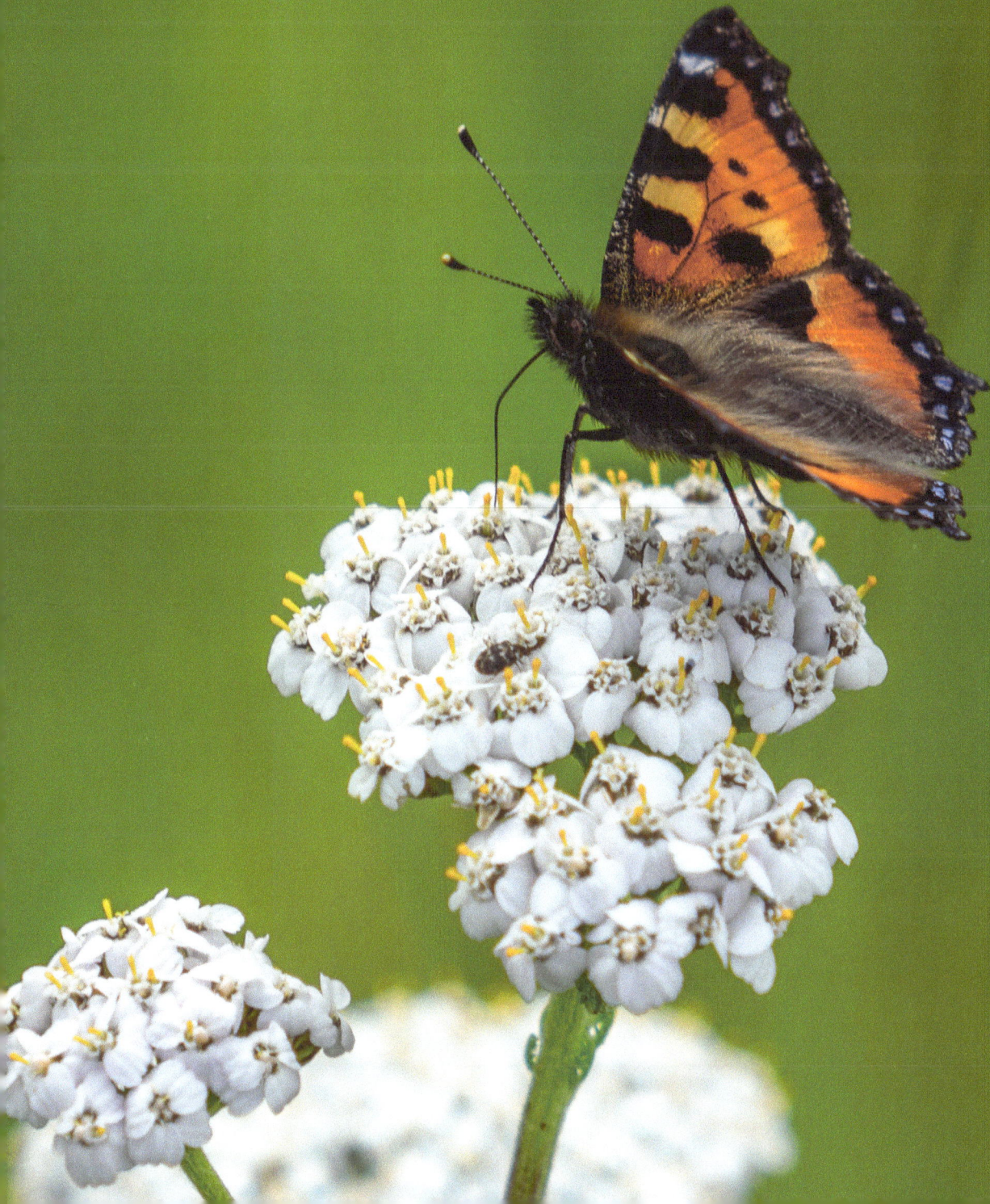

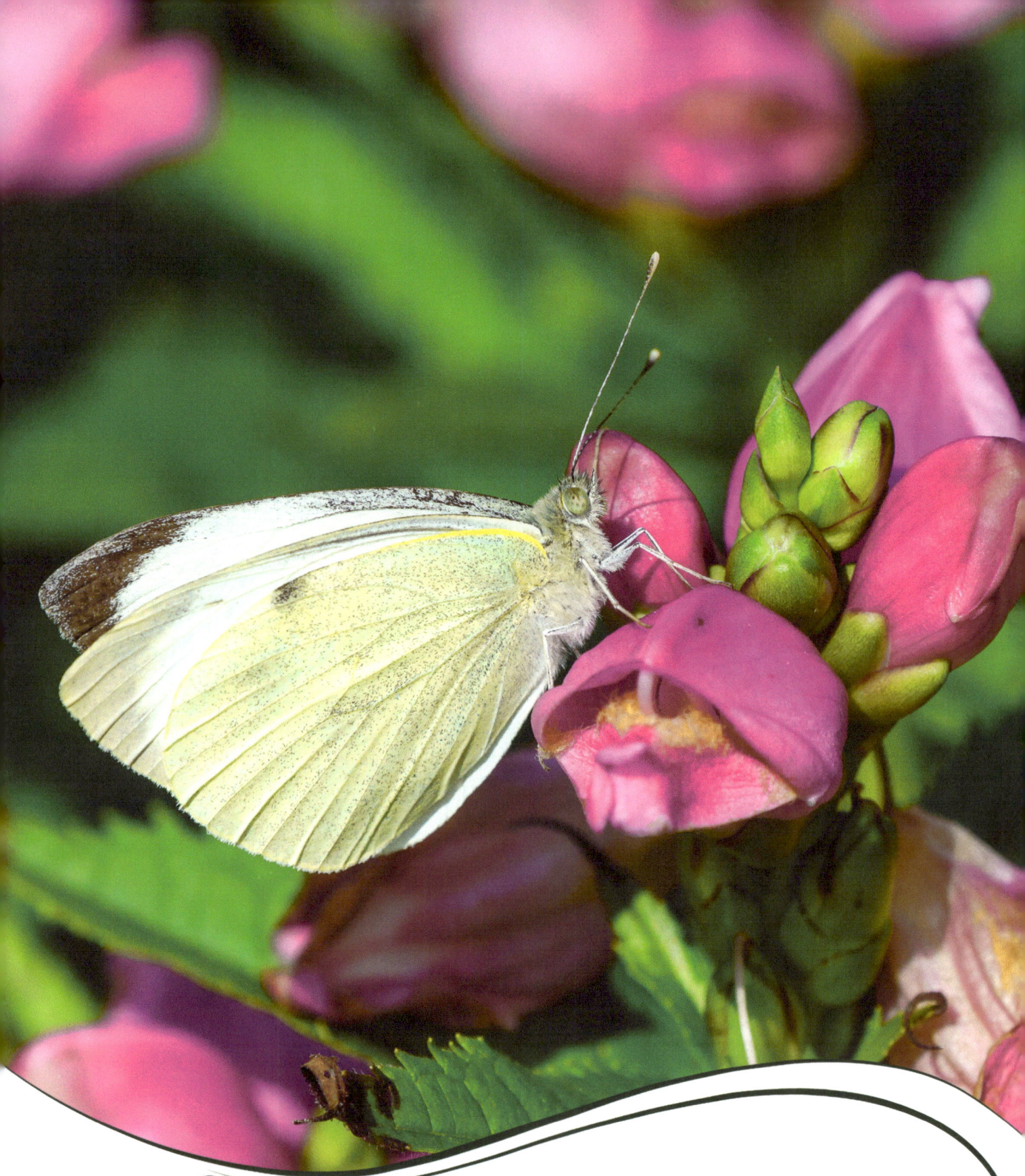

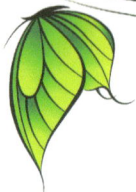

Large White Butterfly

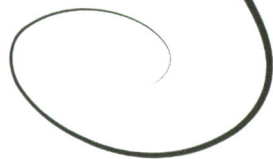

Long-tailed Blue Butterfly

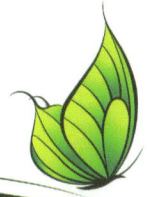

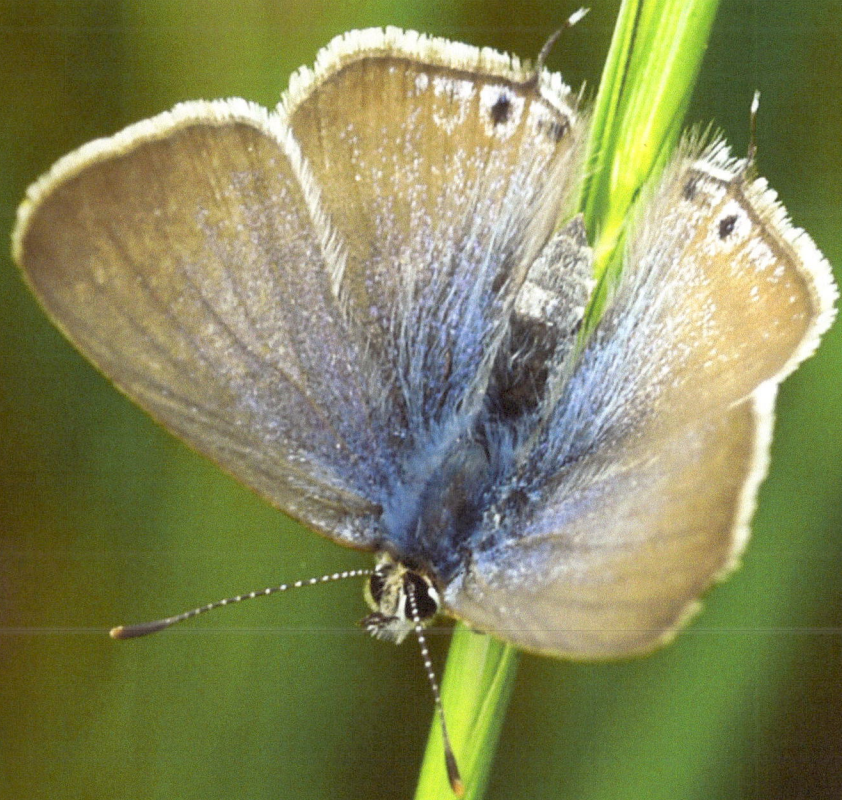

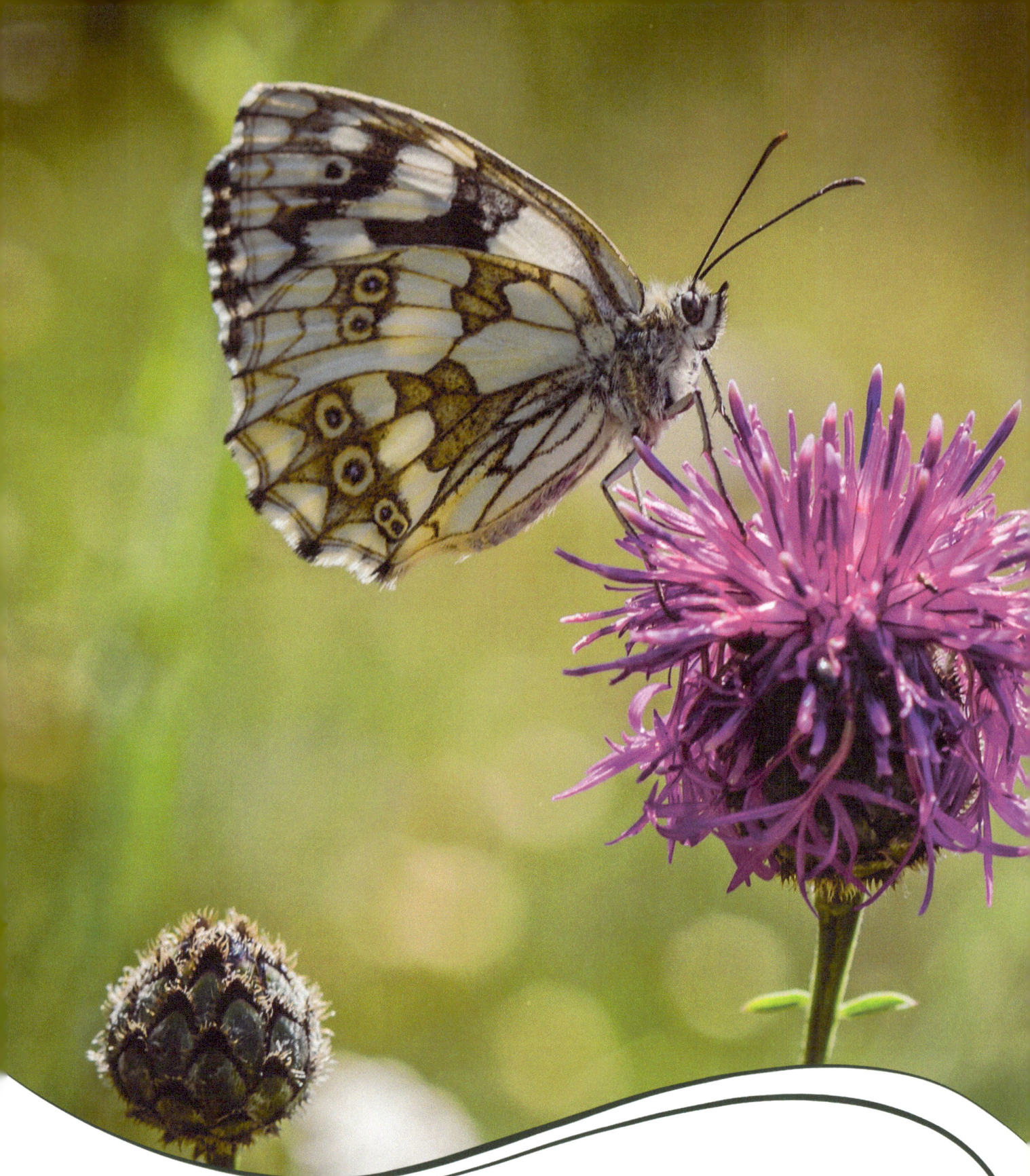

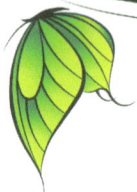

Marbled White
Butterfly

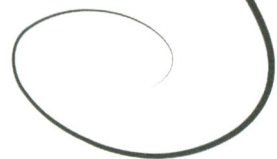

Marsh Fritillary Butterfly

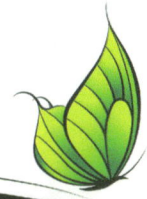

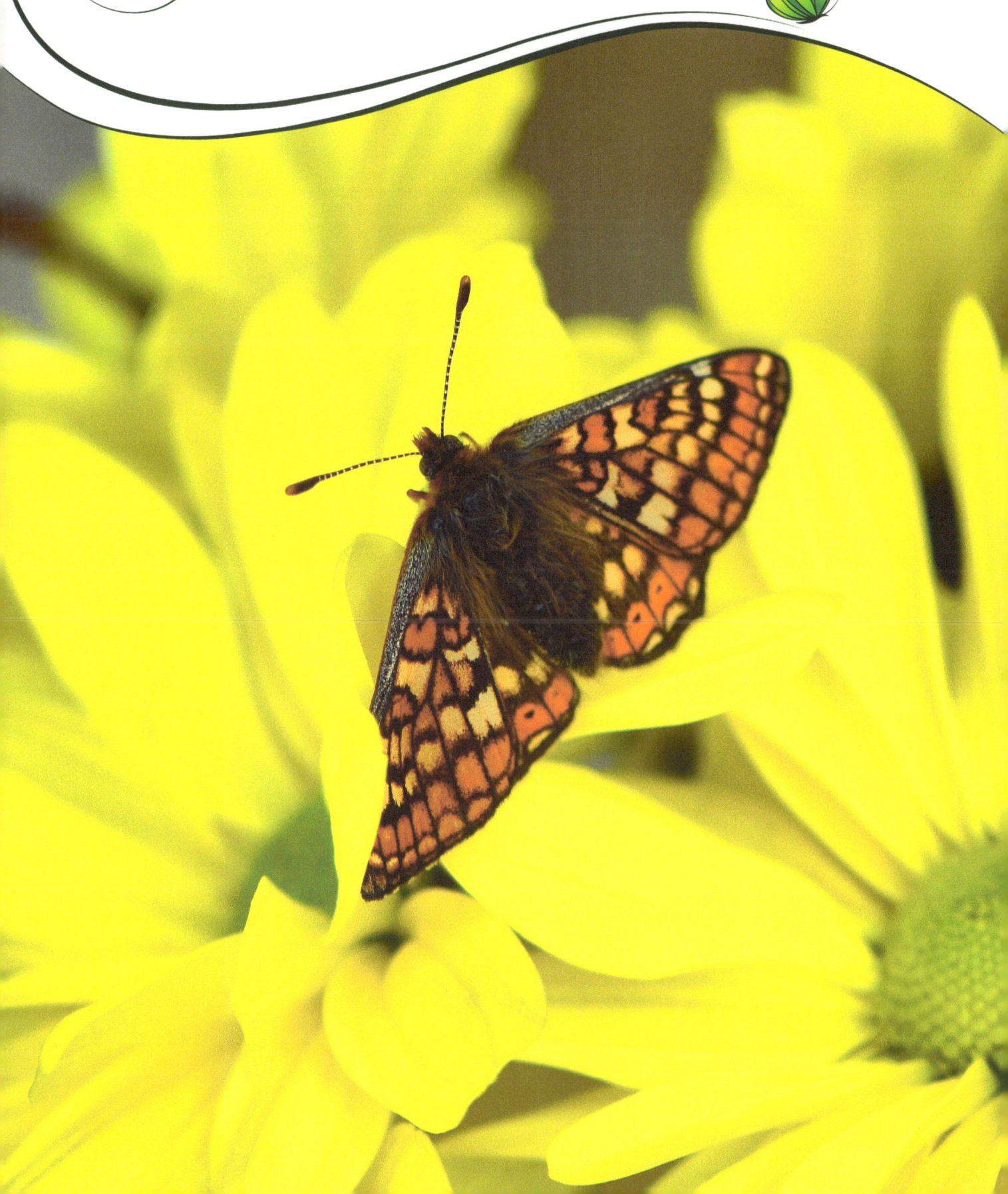

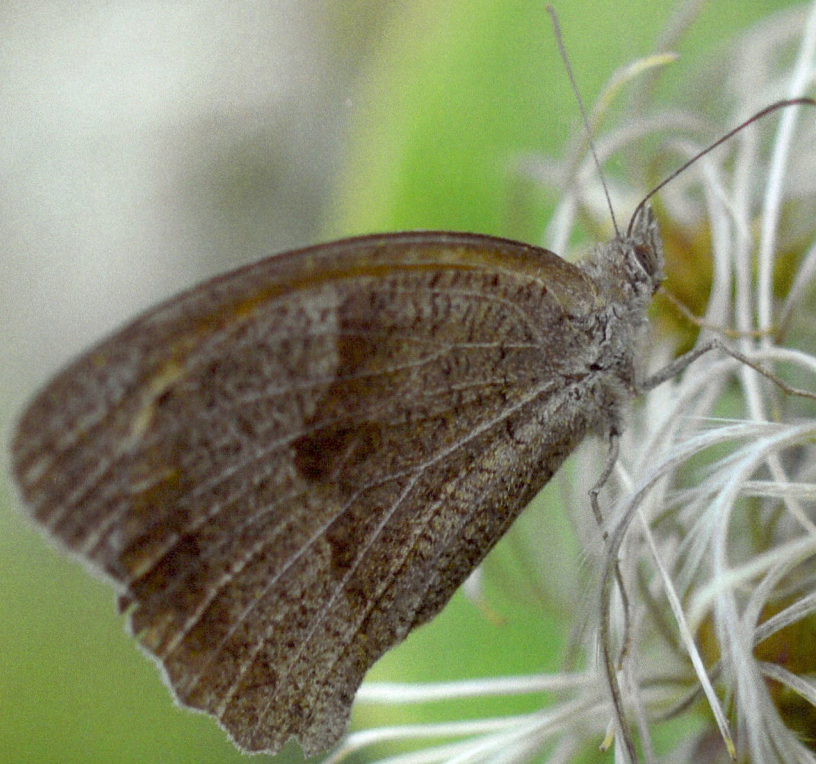

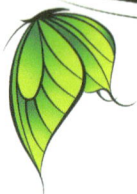

Meadow Brown
Butterfly

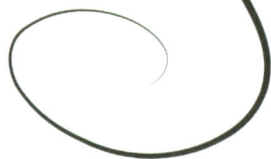

Monarch Butterfly

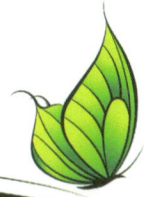

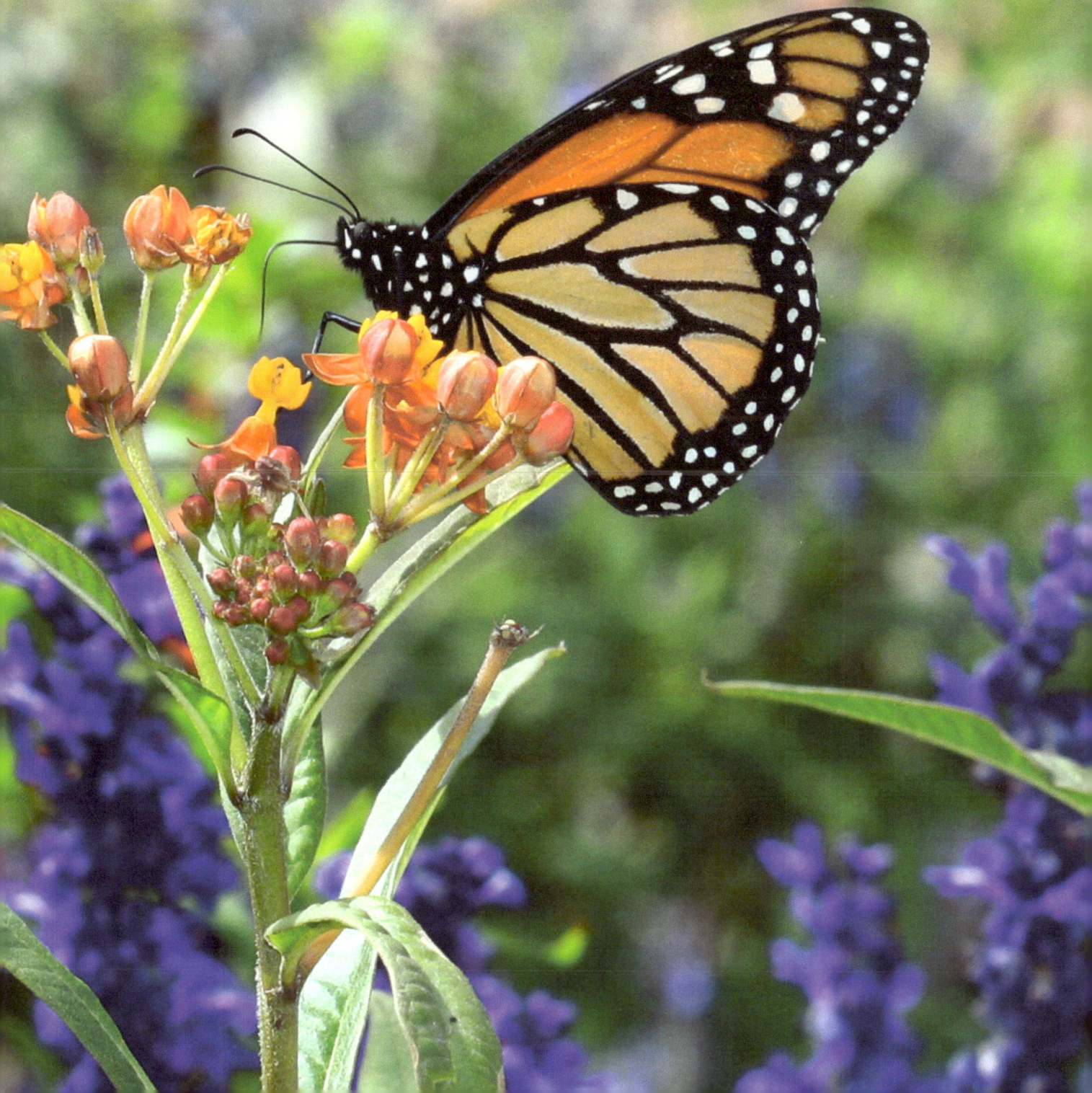

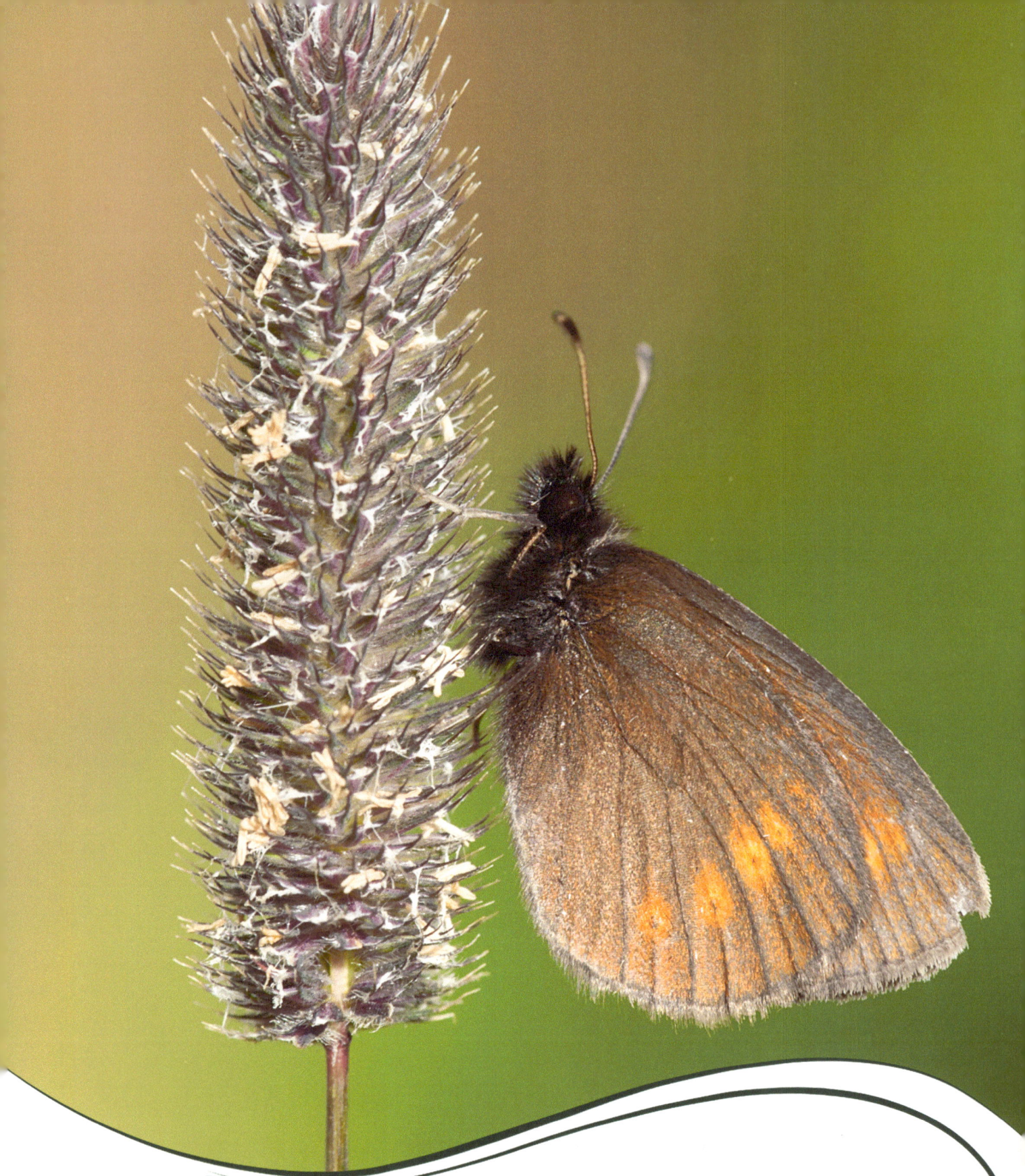

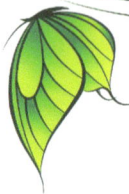

Mountain Ringlet Butterfly

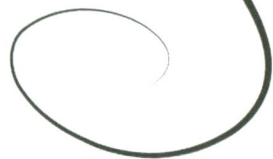

Northern Brown Argus Butterfly

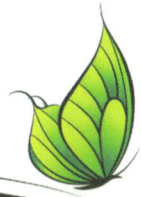

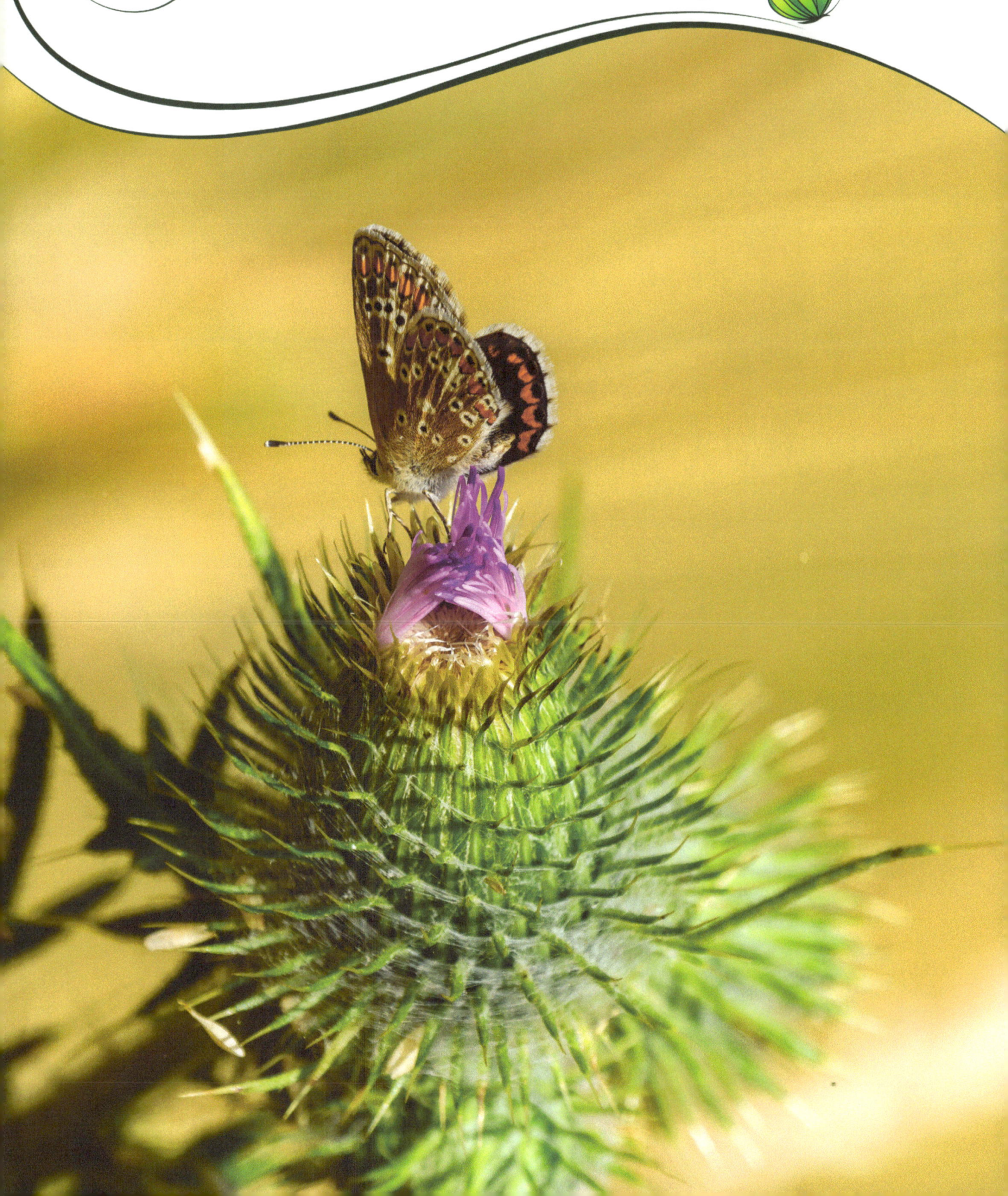

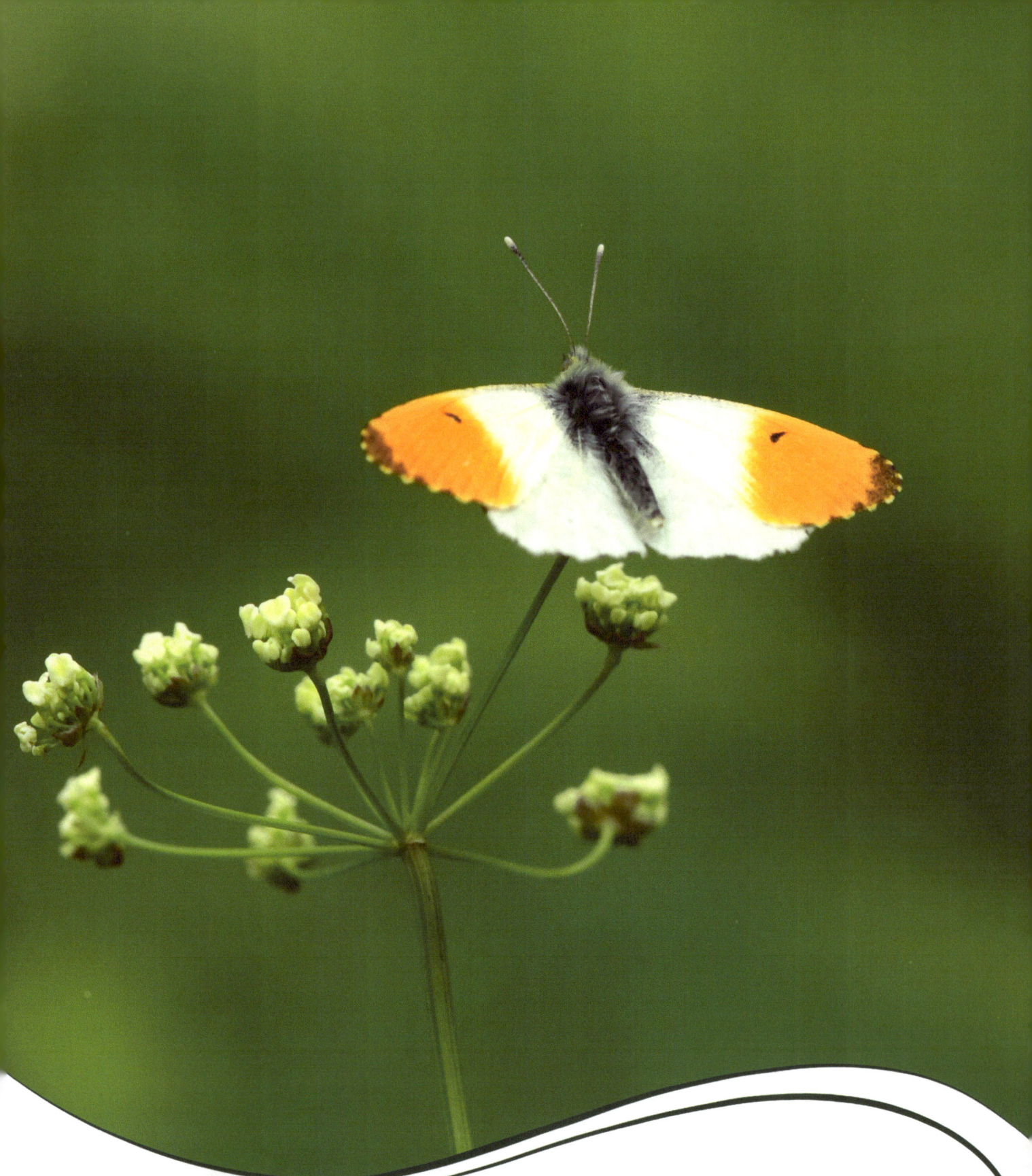

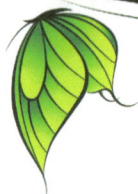

Orange-tip
Butterfly

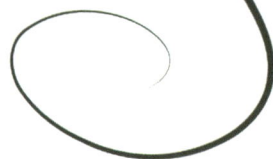

Painted Lady Butterfly

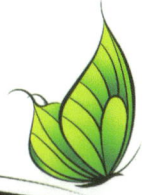

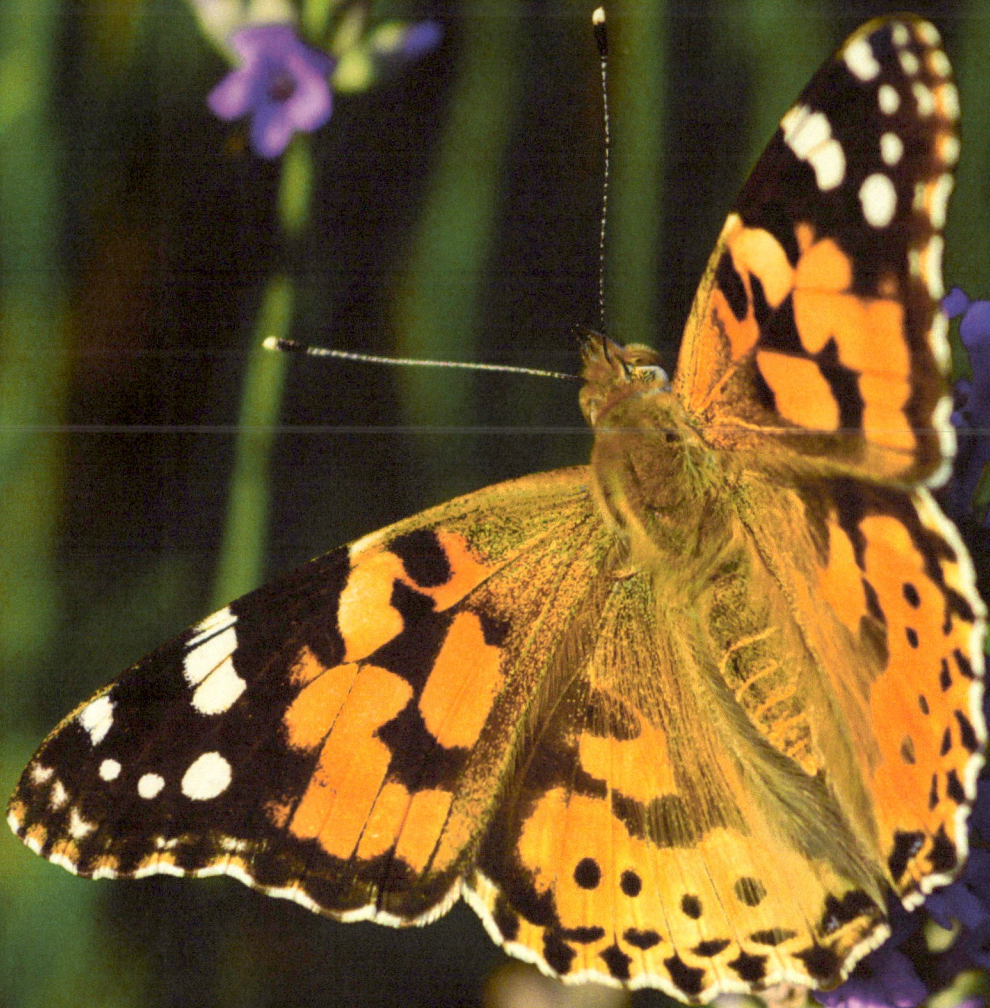

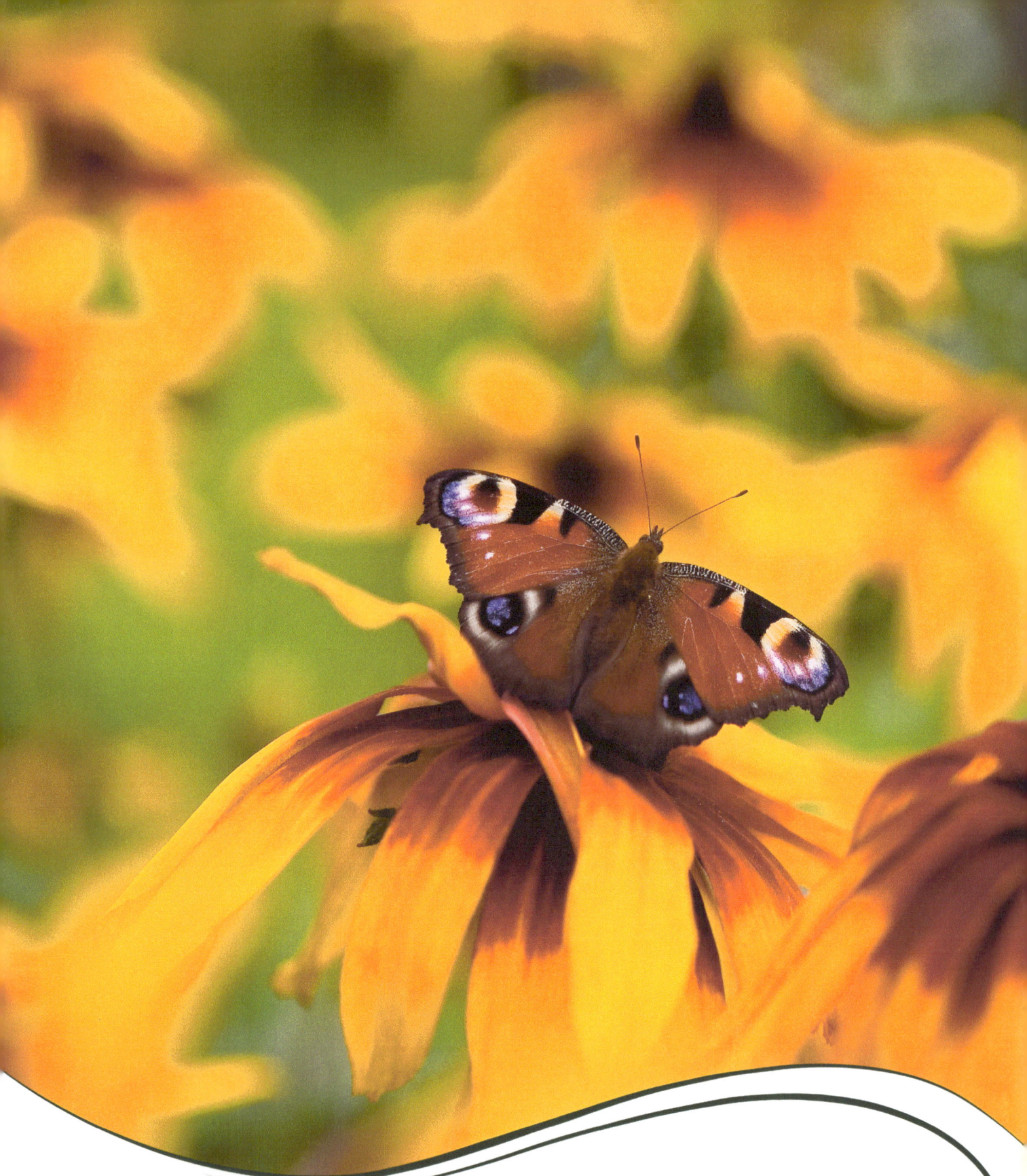

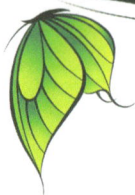

Peacock Butterfly

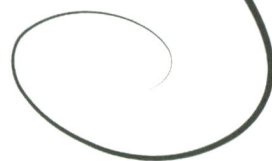

Pearl-bordered Fritillary Butterfly

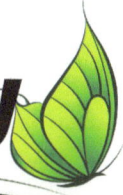

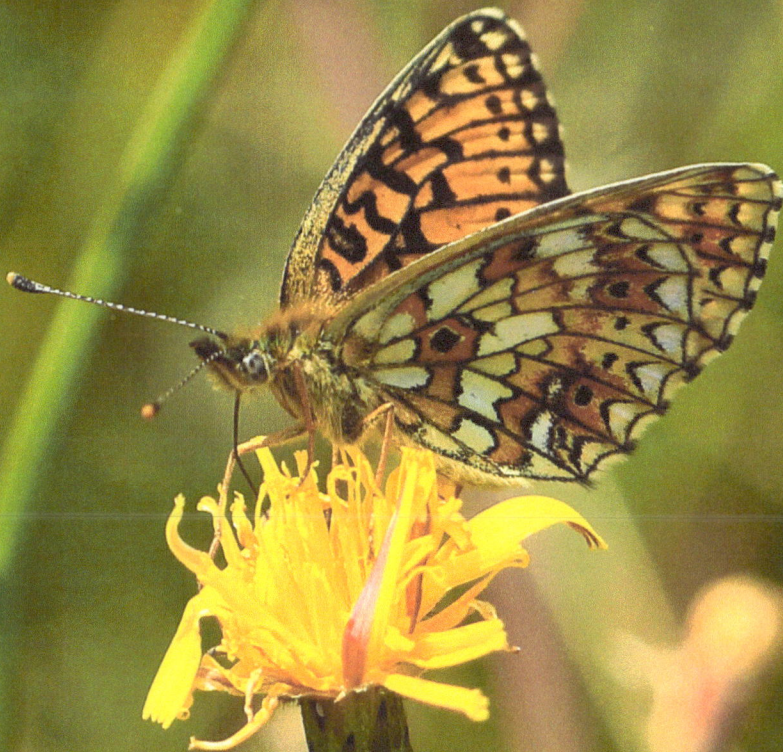

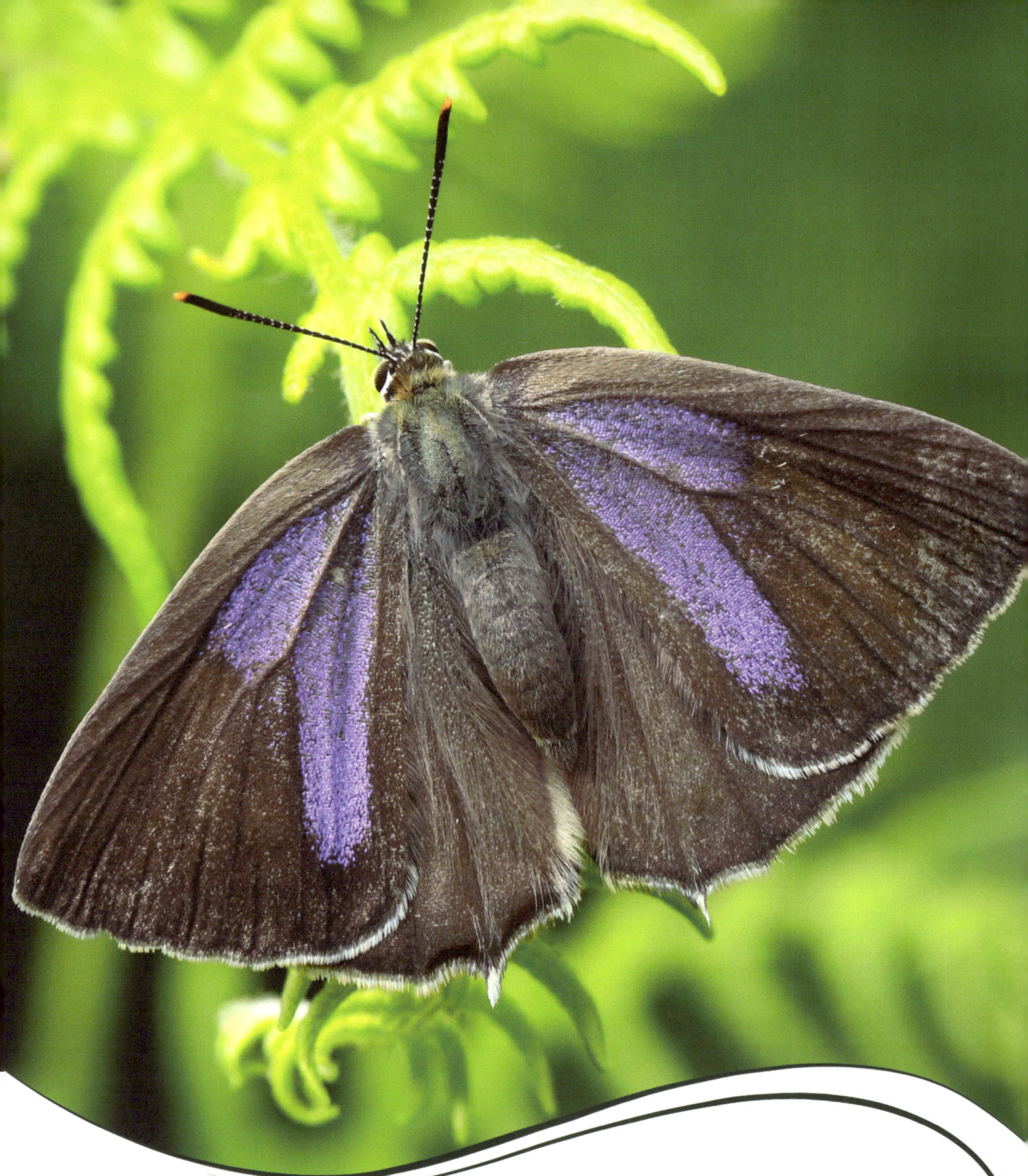

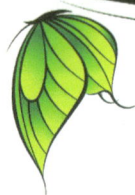

Purple Hairstreak Butterfly

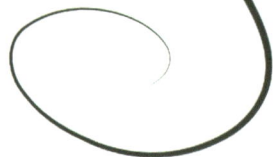

Red Admiral Butterfly

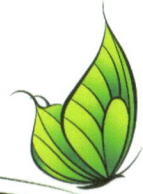

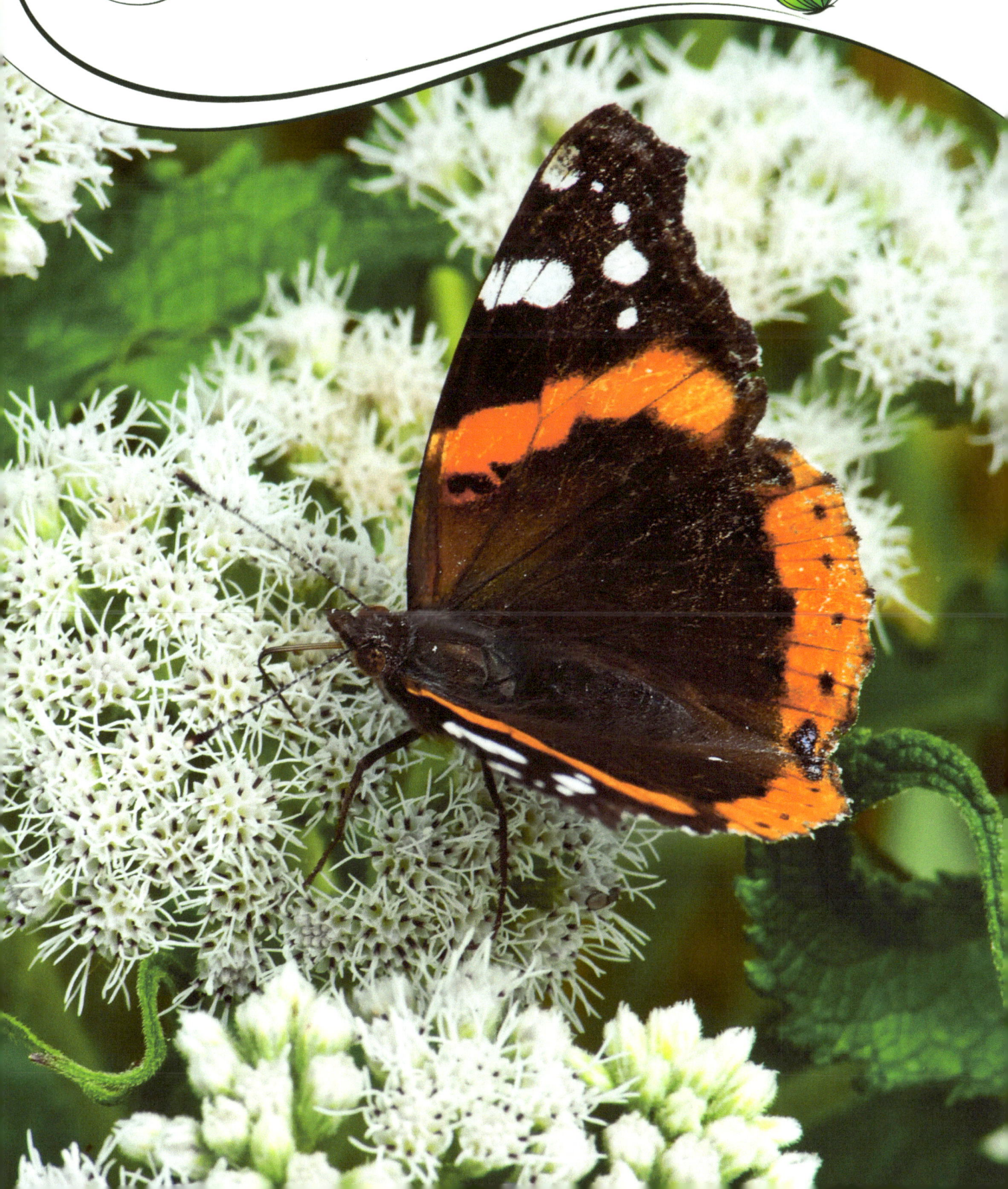

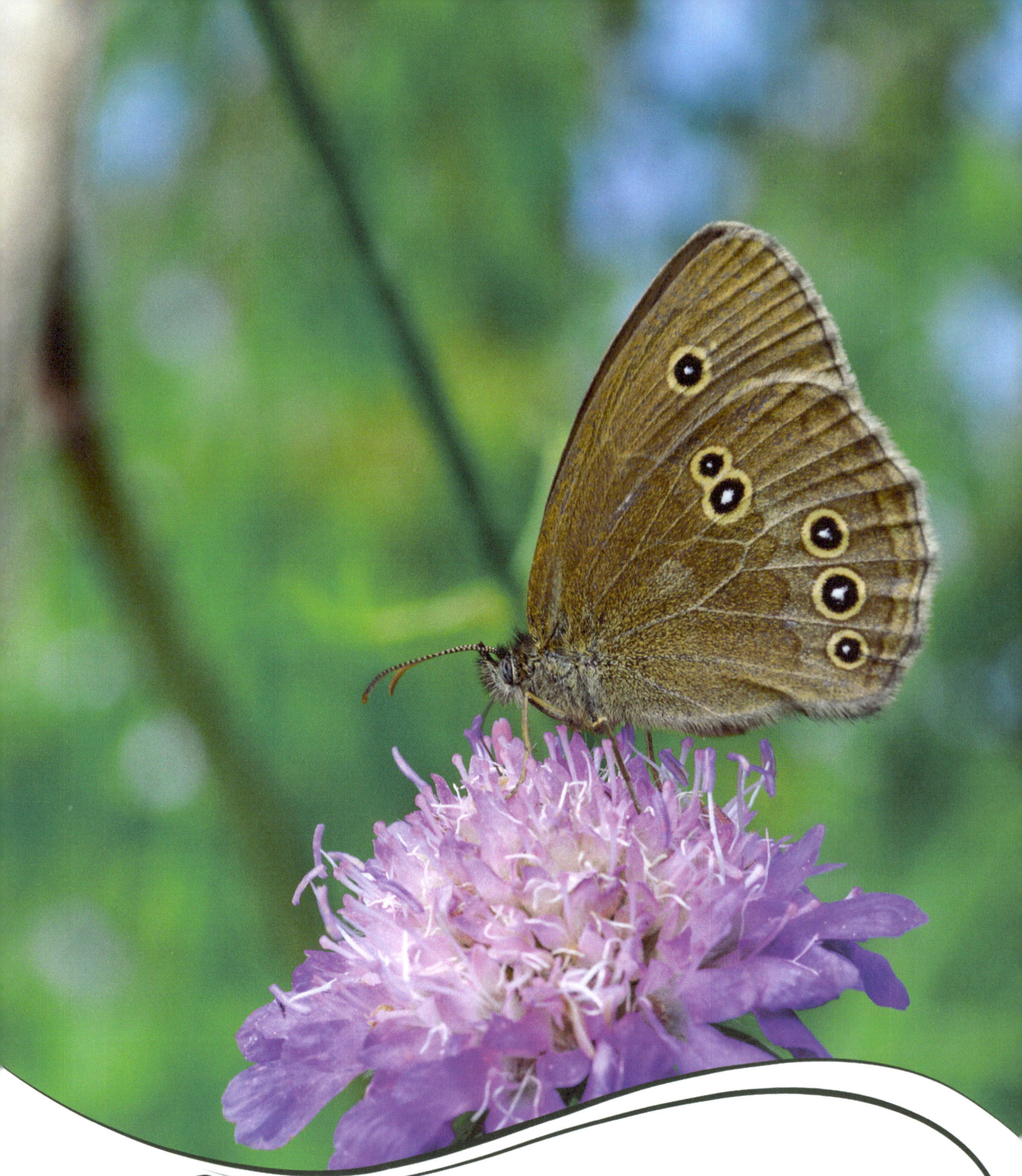

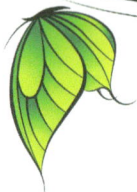

Ringlet
Butterfly

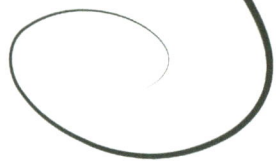

Silver-spotted Skipper Butterfly

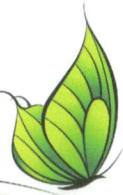

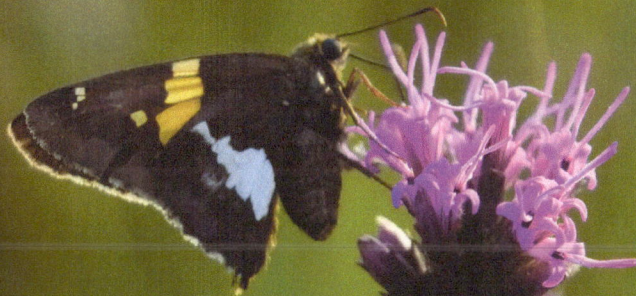

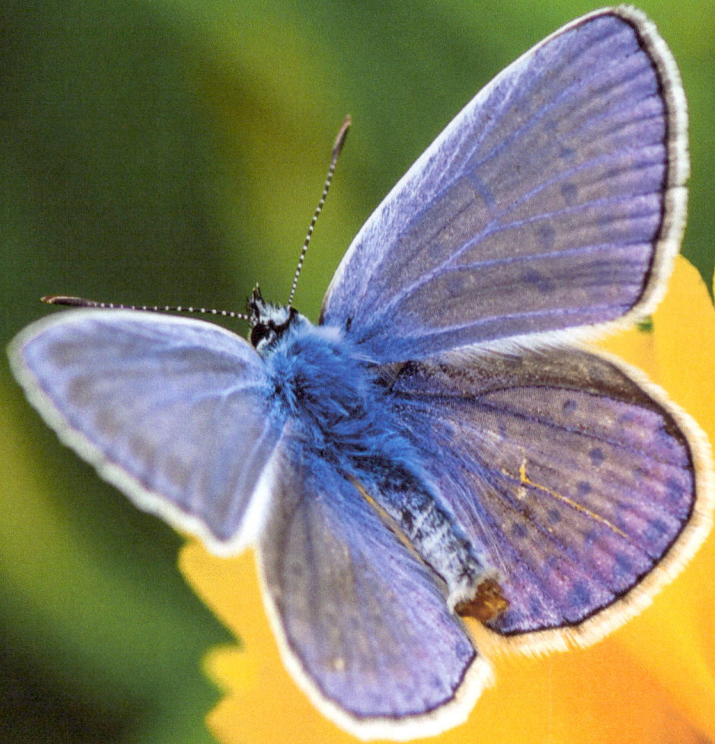

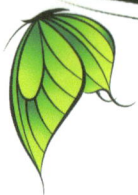

Silver-studded Blue Butterfly

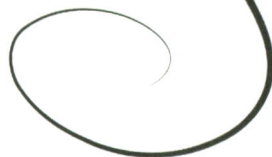

Silver-washed Fritillary Butterfly

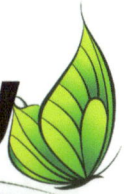

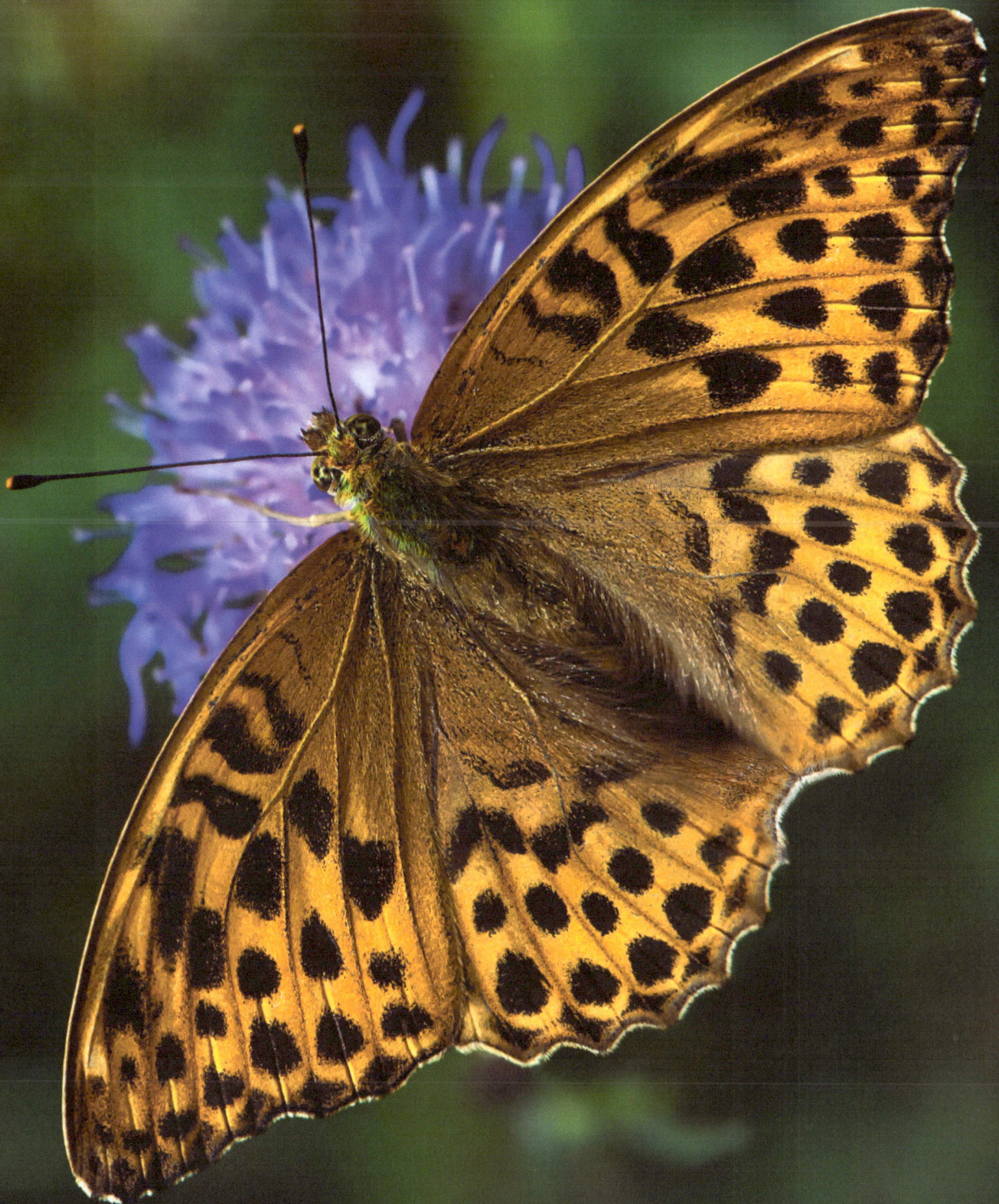

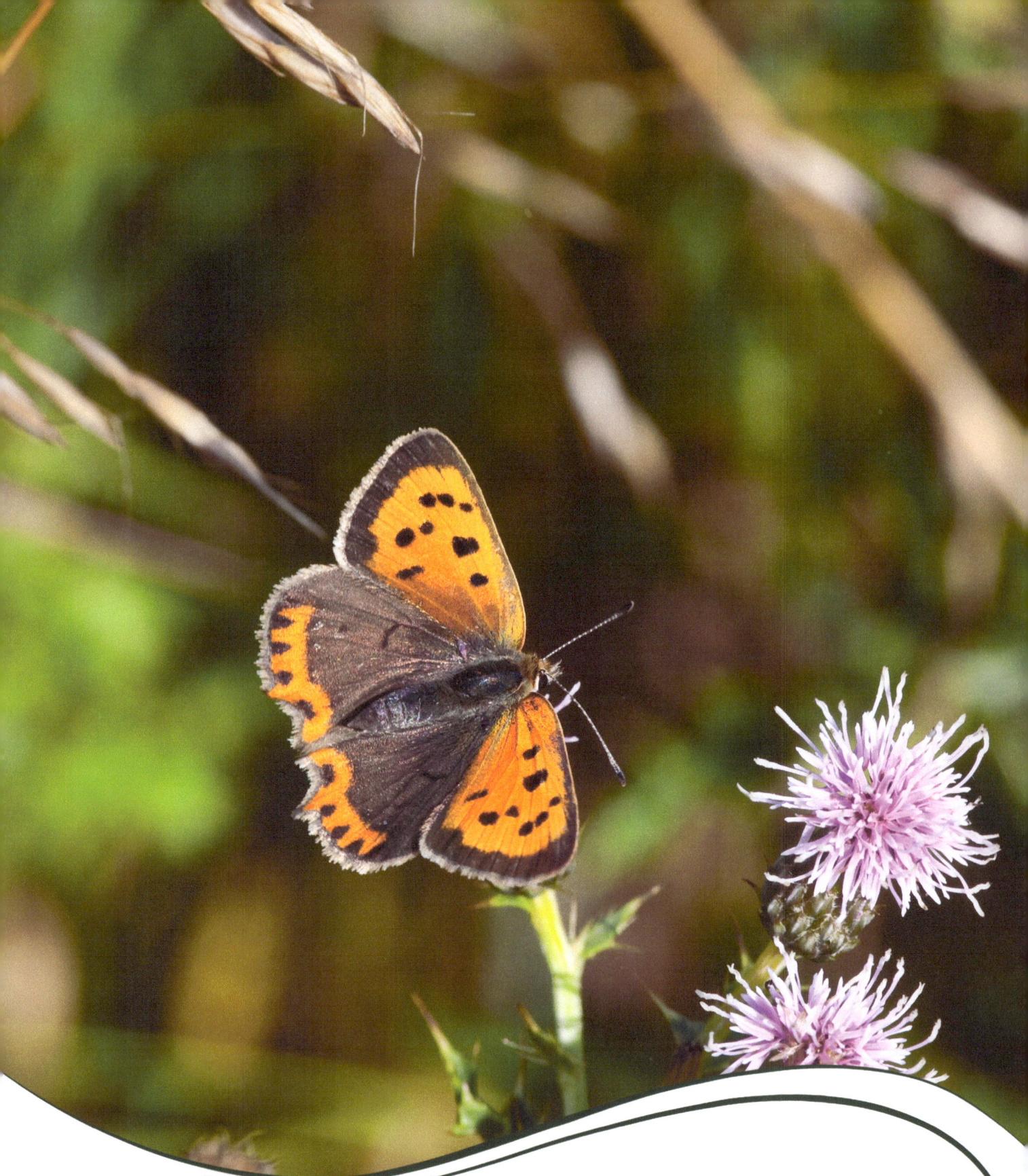

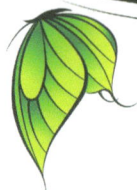

Small Copper Butterfly

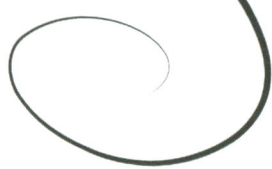

Small Tortoiseshell Butterfly

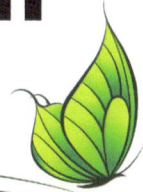

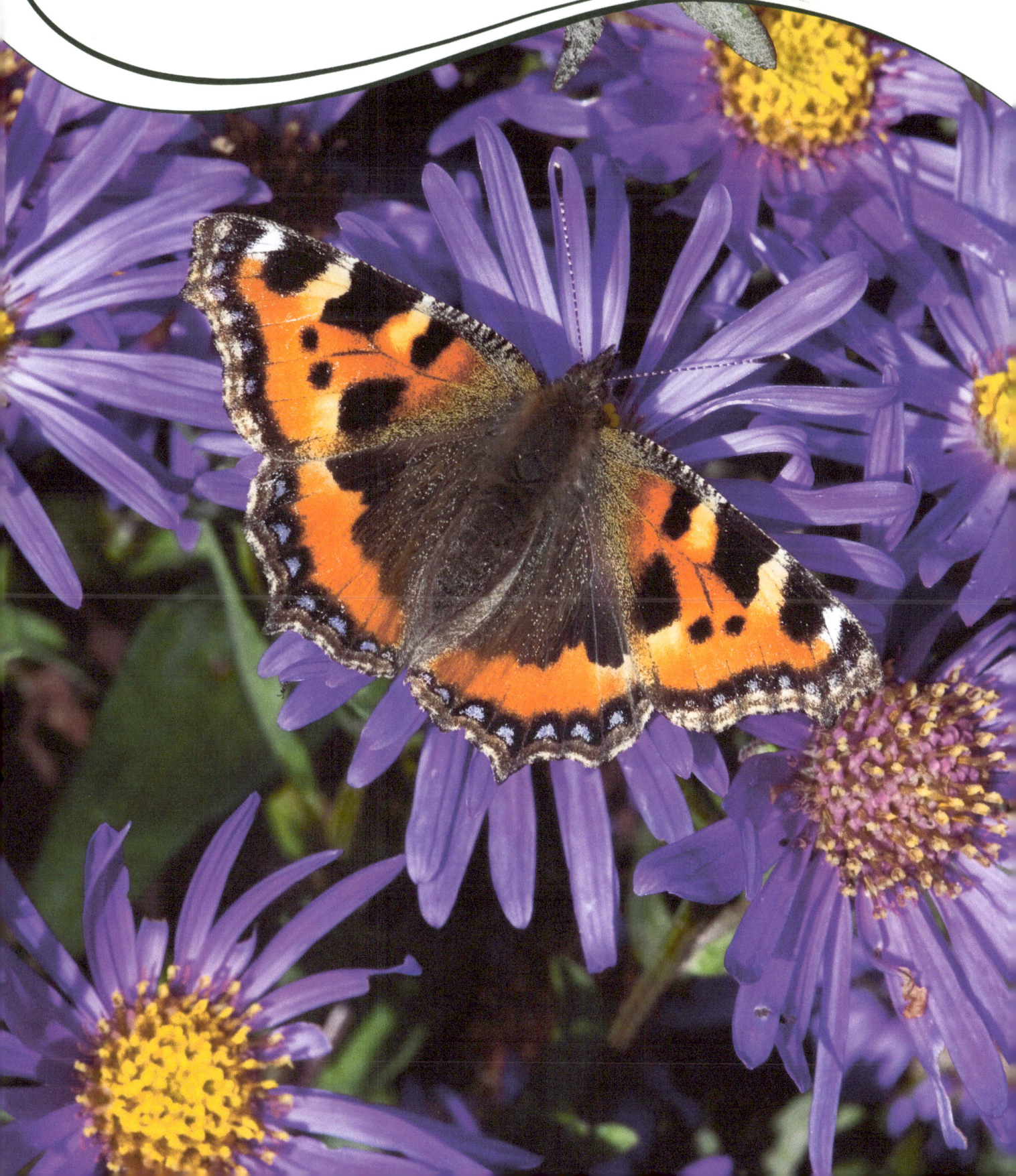

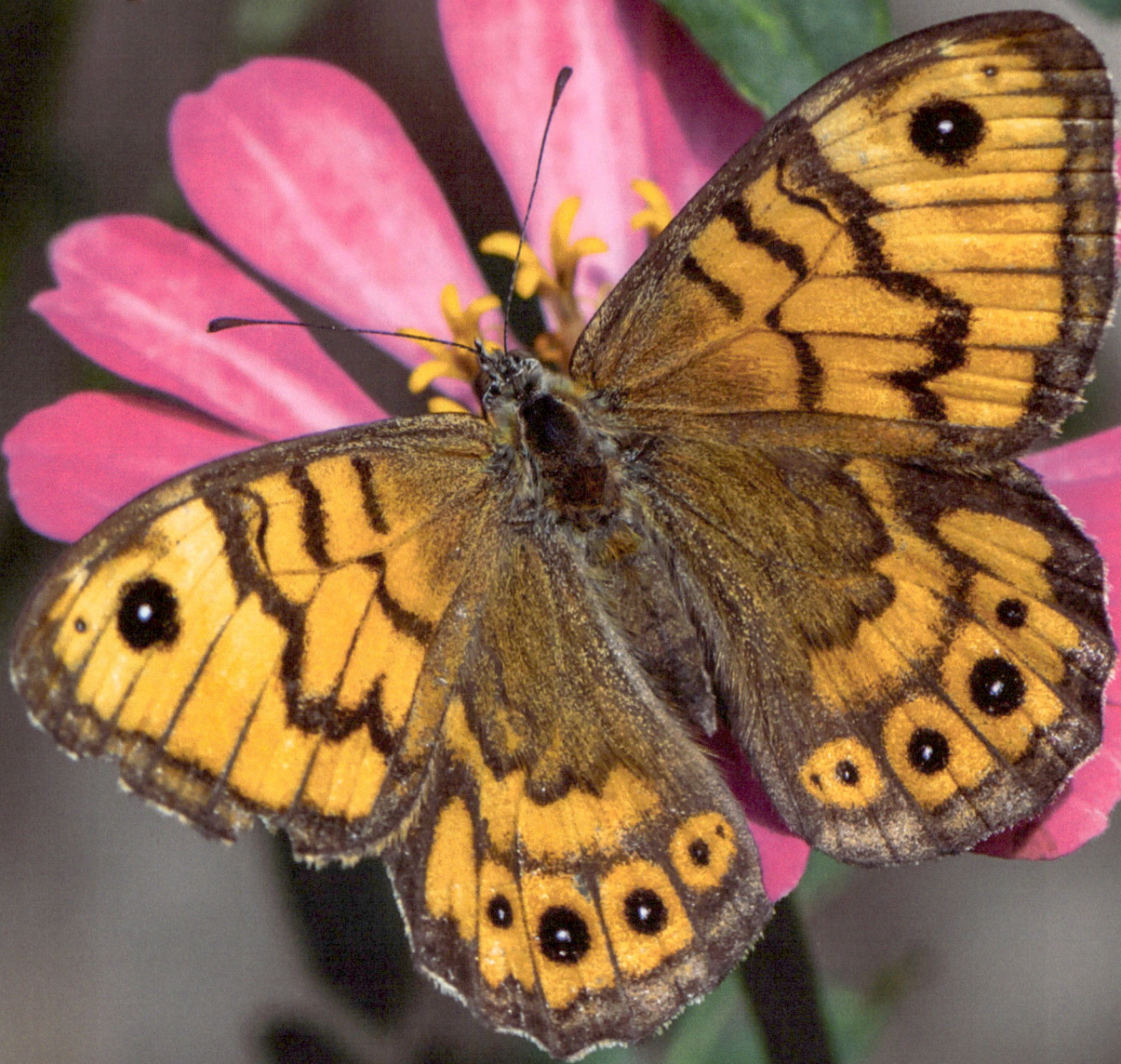

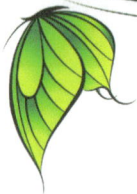

Wall
Butterfly

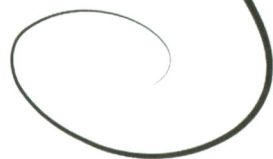

White Admiral Butterfly

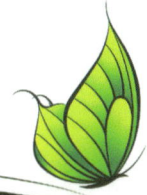

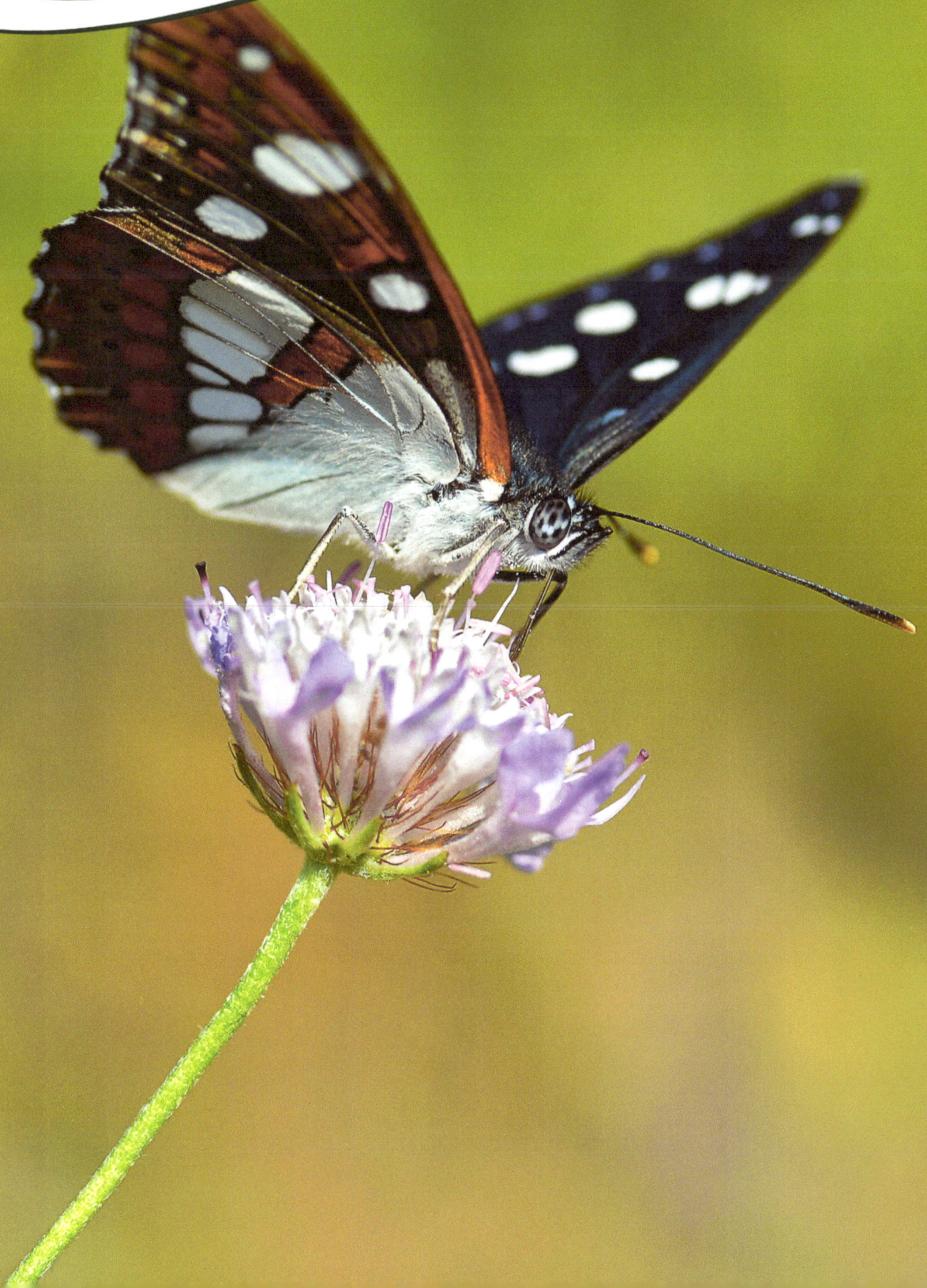

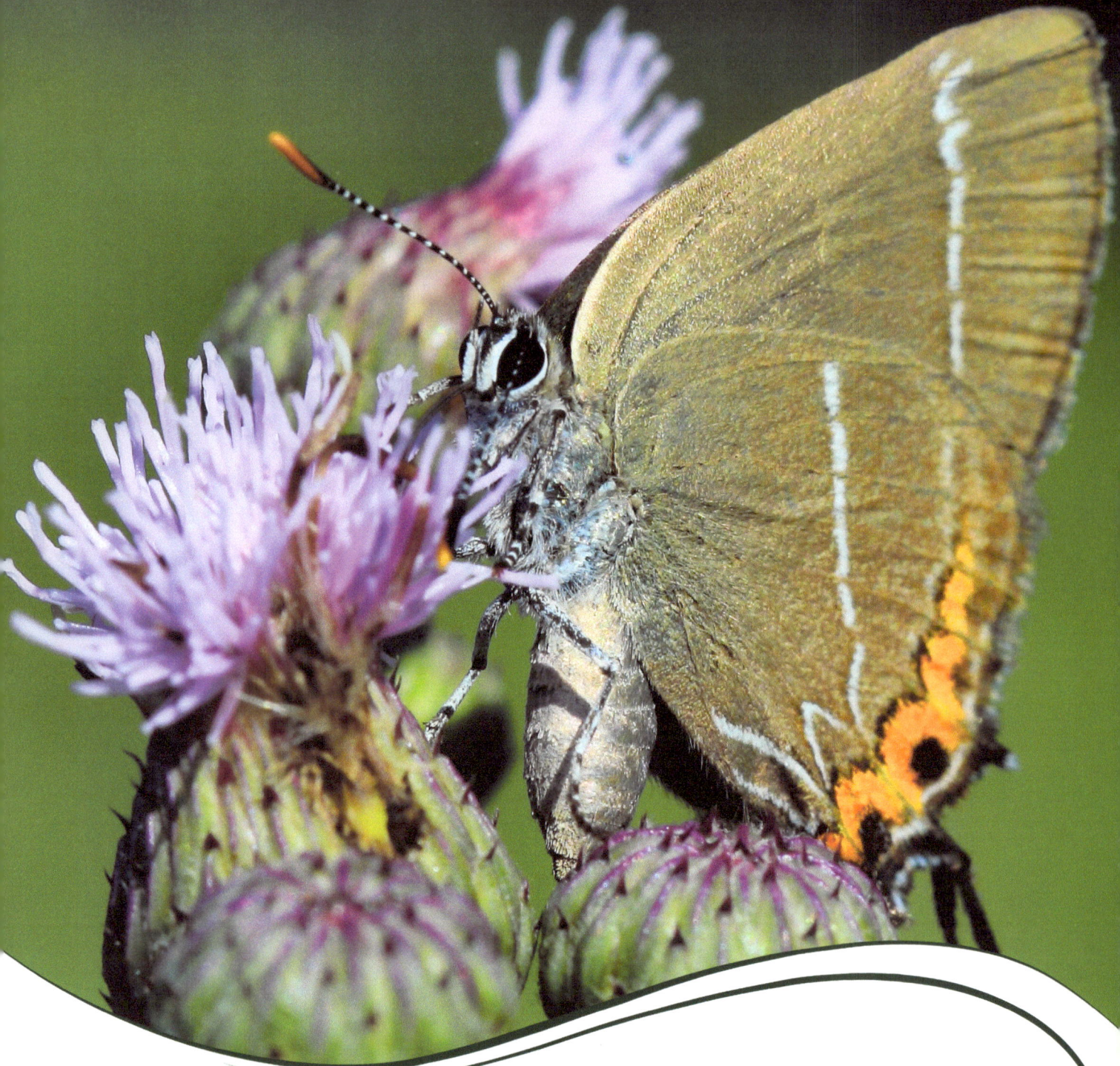

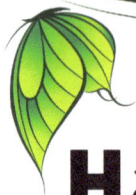

White-letter Hairstreak Butterfly

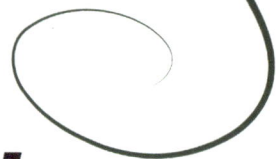

Wood White Butterfly

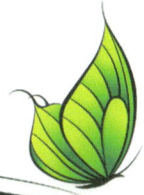

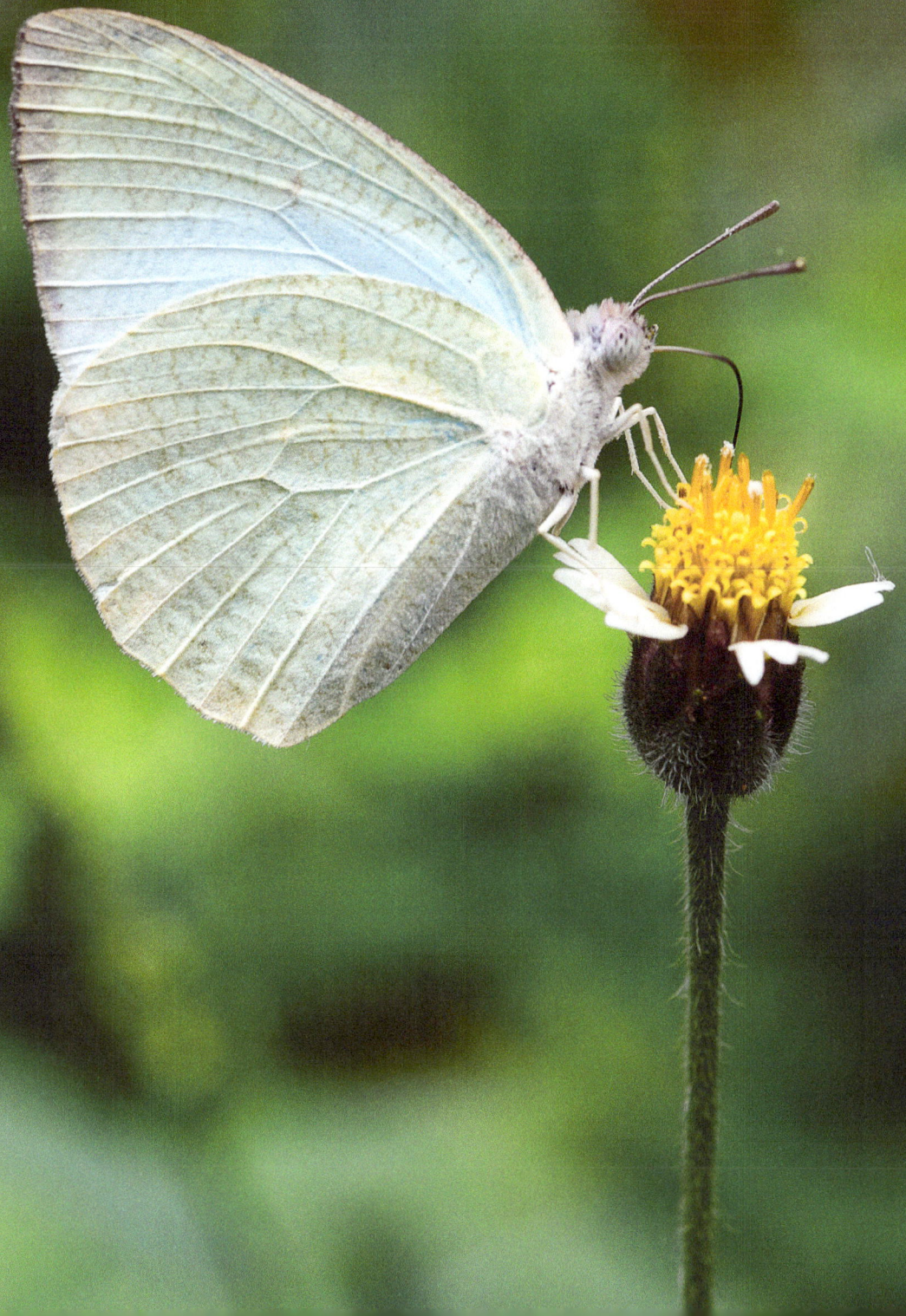

www.ingramcontent.com/pod-product-compliance
Lightning Source LLC
Chambersburg PA
CBHW041544260326
41914CB00015B/1541